Artificial Intelligence - Applications in Medicine and Biology

Edited by Marco Antonio Aceves-Fernandez

Published in London, United Kingdom

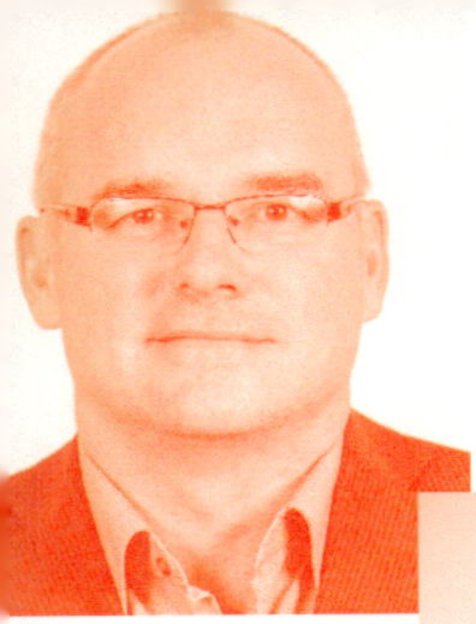
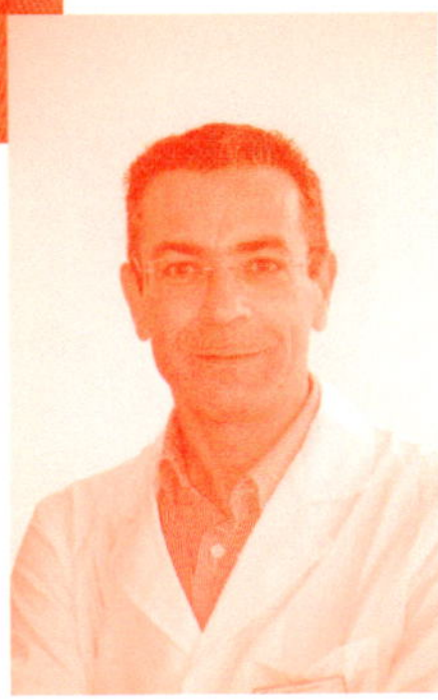
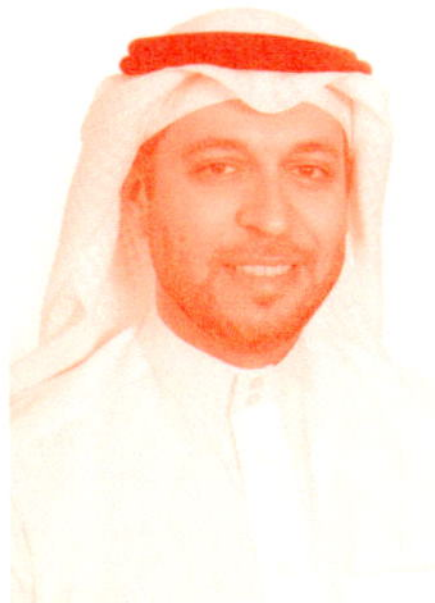
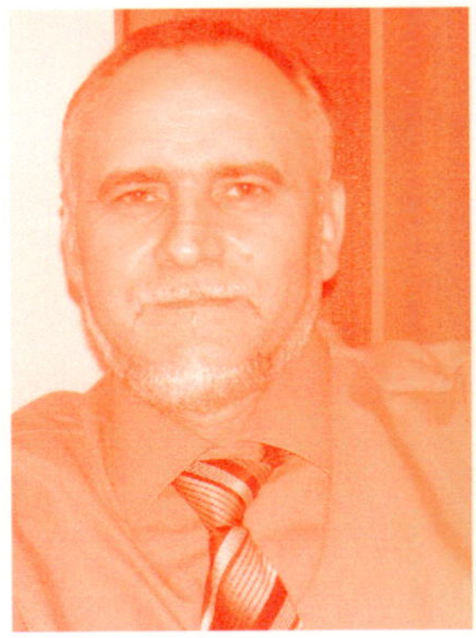
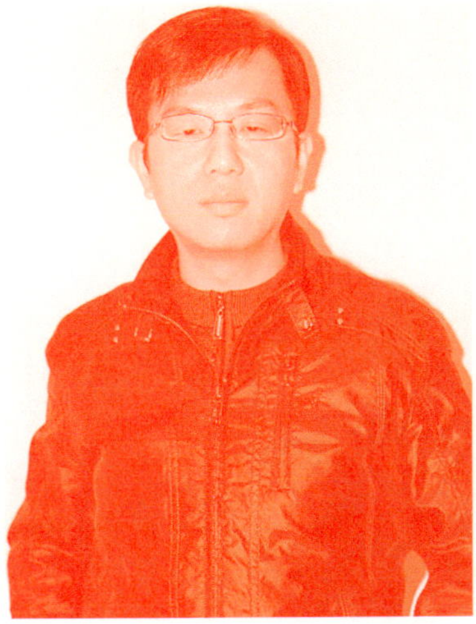
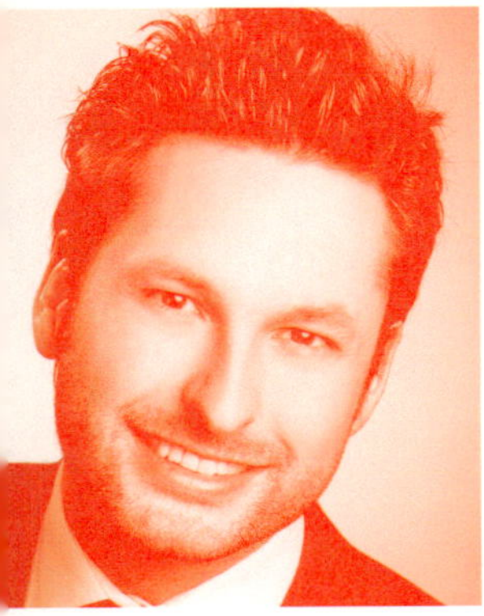
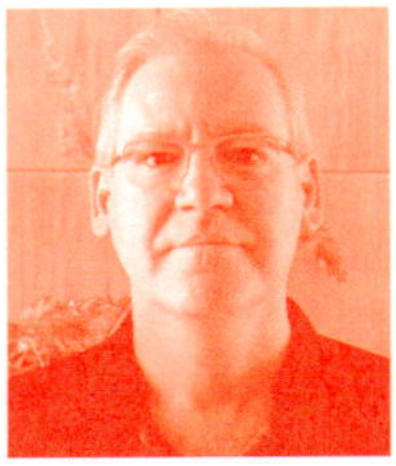

IntechOpen

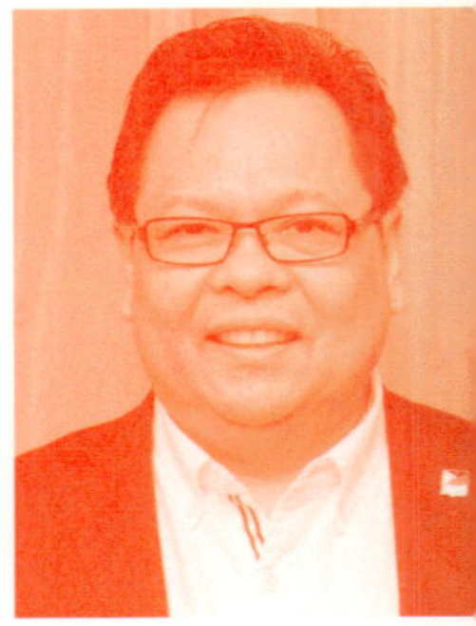
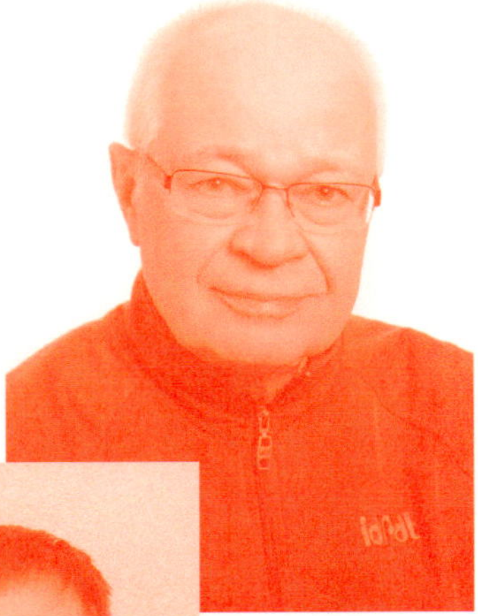
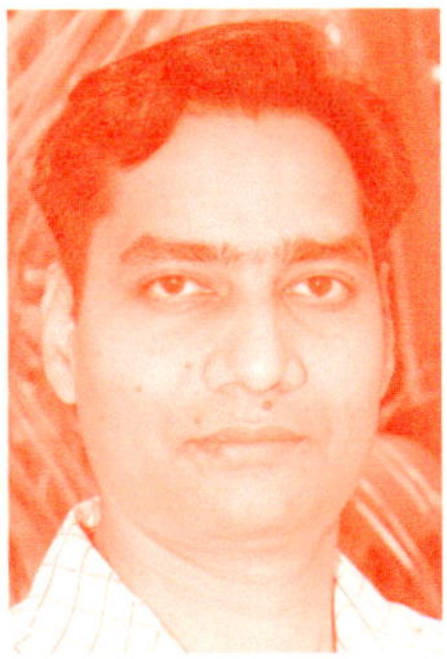
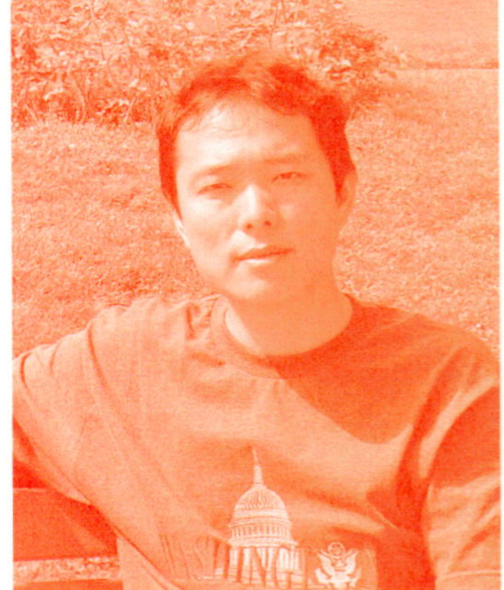
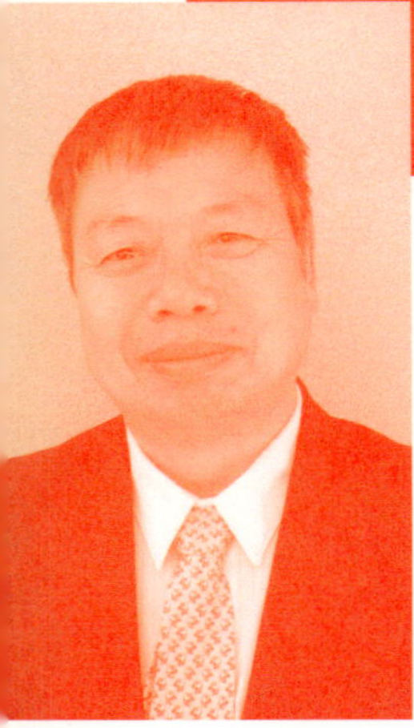
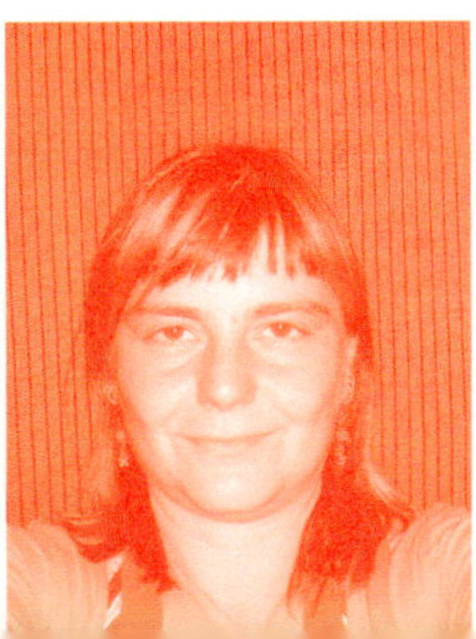

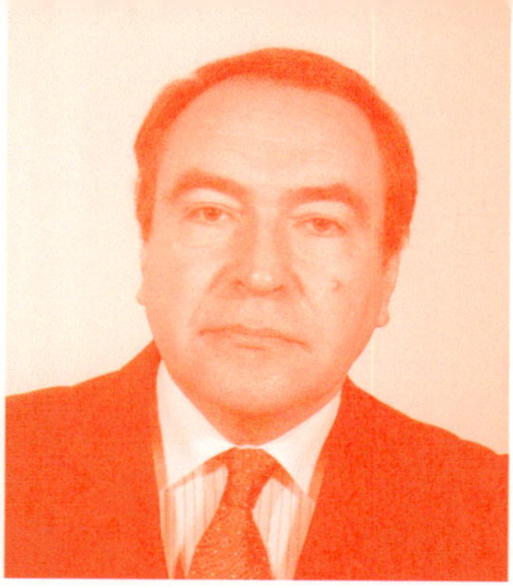
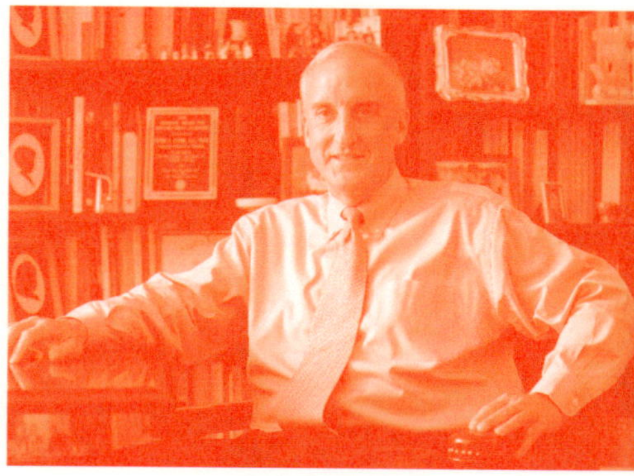
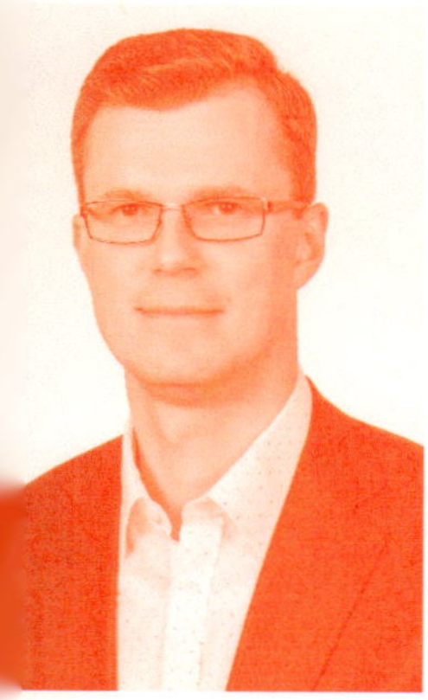
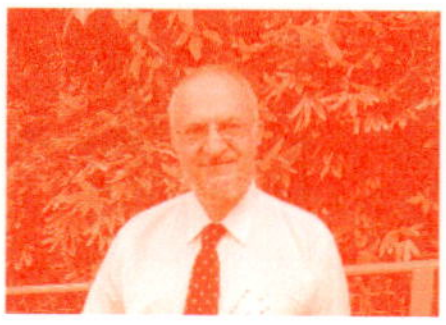
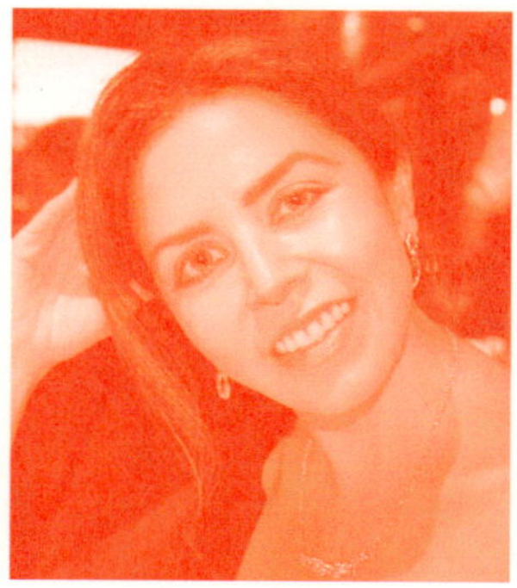

Supporting open minds since 2005

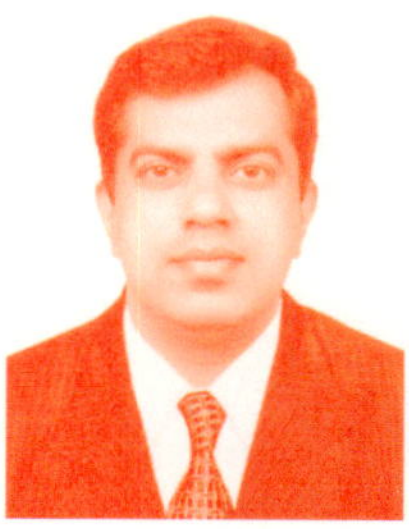
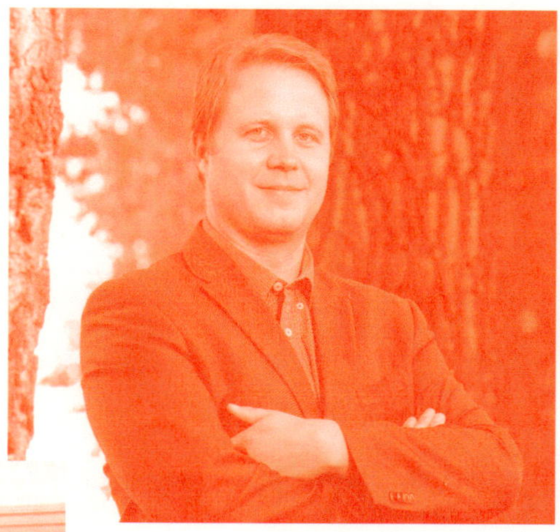
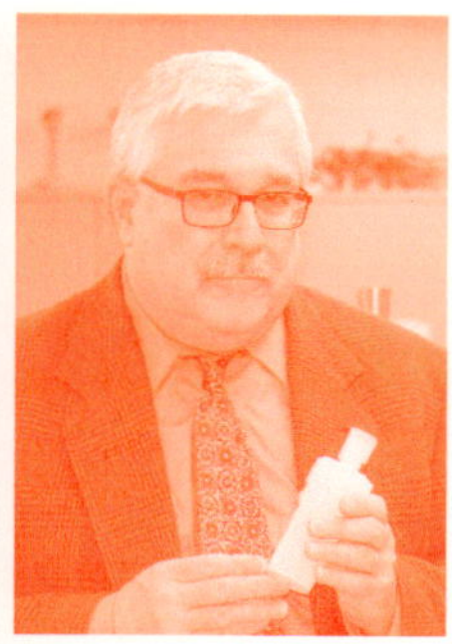
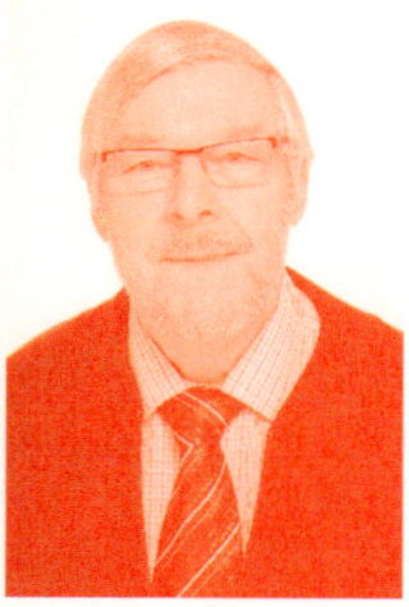
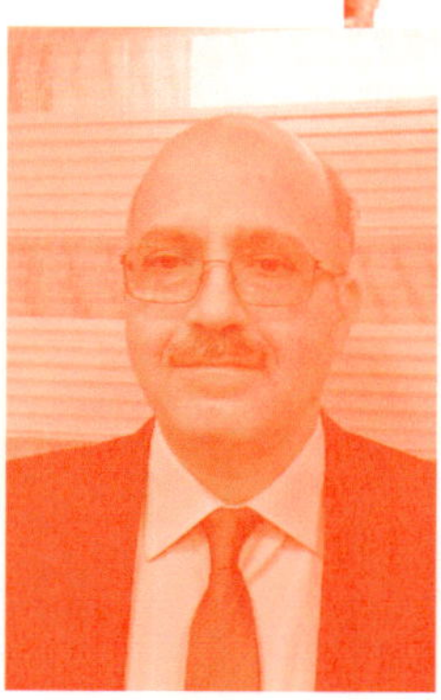
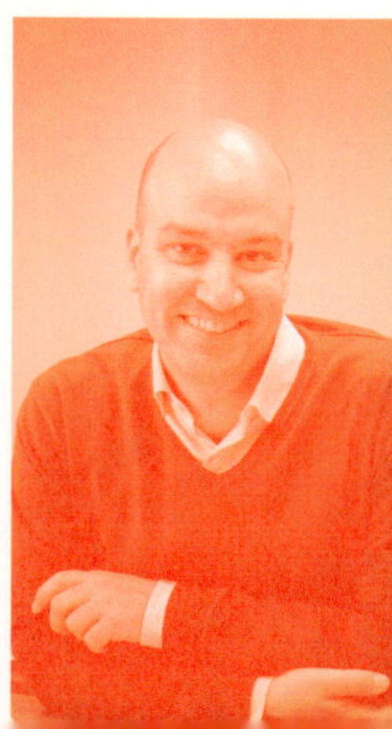
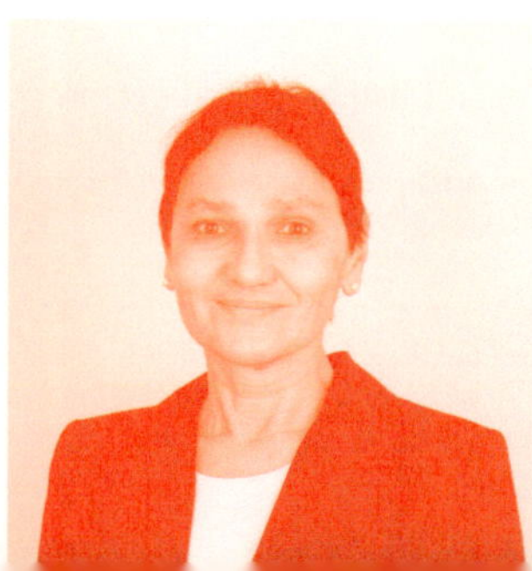

Artificial Intelligence - Applications in Medicine and Biology
http://dx.doi.org/10.5772/intechopen.77536
Edited by Marco Antonio Aceves-Fernandez

Part of IntechOpen Book Series: Artificial Intelligence, Volume 1
Book Series Editor: Marco Antonio Aceves-Fernandez

Contributors
Vei Siang Chan, Farhan Mohamed, Gaston K. Mazandu, Emile R. Chimusa, Irene Kyomugisha, Ephifania Geza, Milaine Seuneu, Bubacarr Bah, Carlos Pedro Gonçalves, Kamran Iqbal, Rajat Emanuel Singh, Gannon White, Jennifer K. Holtz, Joseph Noussa-Yao, Didier Heudes, Patrice Degoulet, Alexander F. I. Osman

First published in London, United Kingdom, 2019 by IntechOpen
IntechOpen is the global imprint of INTECHOPEN LIMITED, registered in England and Wales, registration number: 11086078, The Shard, 25th floor, 32 London Bridge Street
London, SE19SG - United Kingdom
Printed in Croatia

British Library Cataloguing-in-Publication Data
A catalogue record for this book is available from the British Library

Additional hard and PDF copies can be obtained from orders@intechopen.com

Artificial Intelligence - Applications in Medicine and Biology
Edited by Marco Antonio Aceves-Fernandez
p. cm.
Print ISBN 978-1-78984-017-9
Online ISBN 978-1-78984-018-6
eBook (PDF) ISBN 978-1-78984-605-8
ISSN 2633-1403

For EU product safety concerns:
IN TECH d.o.o., Prolaz Marije Krucifikse Kozulić 3, 51000 Rijeka, Croatia, info@intechopen.com or visit our website at intechopen.com.

IntechOpen Book Series

Artificial Intelligence

Volume 1

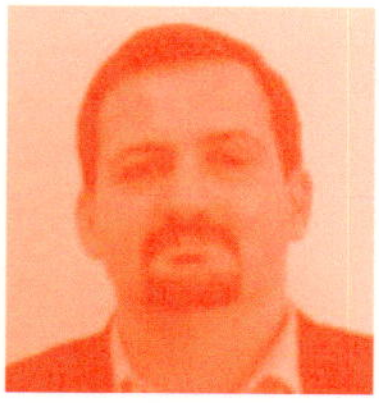

Dr. Marco A. Aceves-Fernandez obtained his BSc (Eng) in Telematics at the Universidad de Colima, Mexico. He obtained both his MSc and PhD at the University of Liverpool, England, in the field of Intelligent Systems. He is full professor at the Universidad Autonoma de Queretaro, Mexico. He has been a member of the National System of Researchers (SNI) since 2009. Dr. Aceves-Fernandez has published more than 80 research papers as well as a number of book chapters and congress papers. He has contributed to more than 20 funded research projects, both academic and industrial, on artificial intelligence and its applications in fields such as environmental, biomedical, automotive, aviation, consumer, and robotics. He is also honorary president at the Mexican Association of Embedded Systems (AMESE), a senior member of the Institute of Electrical and Electronics Engineers (IEEE), and a board member for many institutions and associations. His research interests include intelligent and embedded systems.

Book Series Editor and Editor of Volume 1: Marco A. Aceves-Fernandez
Universidad Autonoma de Queretaro, Mexico

Scope of the Series

Artificial Intelligence (AI) is a rapidly developing multidisciplinary research area that aims to solve increasingly complex problems. In today´s highly integrated world, AI promises to become a robust and powerful mean for obtaining solutions to previously unsolvable problems. This book series is intended for researchers and students alike, as well as all those interested in this fascinating field and its applications, in particular in areas related to the topics on which it is focused.

Contents

Preface

Artificial intelligence (AI) is taking on an increasingly important role in our society today. In the early days, machines fulfilled only manual activities. Nowadays, these machines extend their capabilities to cognitive tasks as well. And now AI is poised to make a huge contribution to medical and biological applications.

Scientists and doctors alike are fascinated by the potential of AI. As computer systems become increasingly more intelligent and capable of storing and processing vast amounts of information, interest in AI has started to grow as well. For example, AI has great potential for use in medical equipment, disease diagnosis and prognosis, medical care, healthcare infrastructure, and image and video processing, among others. Much recent scientific research has focused on using accurate, reliable, and robust intelligent systems to accurately diagnose and predict patterns of disease.

The ability of AI to make informed decisions, learn and perceive the environment, and predict certain behavior, among its many other skills, makes this application of paramount importance in today's world.

This book is organized into the following sections:

1. Machine Learning Applications

2. Image Processing in Medicine and Biology

3. Emerging Paradigms of Machine Learning

This work will be of interest to students and researchers alike, as it comprises quality research contributions with a number of different applications.

Marco Antonio Aceves-Fernandez, Ph.D.
Universidad Autonoma de Queretaro,
Mexico

Section 1

Machine Learning Applications

Chapter 1

Designing Data-Driven Learning Algorithms: A Necessity to Ensure Effective Post-Genomic Medicine and Biomedical Research

Gaston K. Mazandu, Irene Kyomugisha, Ephifania Geza, Milaine Seuneu, Bubacarr Bah and Emile R. Chimusa

Abstract

Advances in sequencing technology have significantly contributed to shaping the area of genetics and enabled the identification of genetic variants associated with complex traits through genome-wide association studies. This has provided insights into genetic medicine, in which case, genetic factors influence variability in disease and treatment outcomes. On the other side, the missing or hidden heritability has suggested that the host quality of life and other environmental factors may also influence differences in disease risk and drug/treatment responses in genomic medicine, and orient biomedical research, even though this may be highly constrained by genetic capabilities. It is expected that combining these different factors can yield a paradigm-shift of personalized medicine and lead to a more effective medical treatment. With existing "big data" initiatives and high-performance computing infrastructures, there is a need for data-driven learning algorithms and models that enable the selection and prioritization of relevant genetic variants (post-genomic medicine) and trigger effective translation into clinical practice. In this chapter, we survey and discuss existing machine learning algorithms and post-genomic analysis models supporting the process of identifying valuable markers.

Keywords: learning algorithms, machine learning, genome-wide association study, genomic medicine, biomedical research, post-genomic analysis

1. Introduction

Advancements in the human deoxyribonucleic acid (DNA) microarray and genome sequencing technology have resulted in an exponential growth of publicly available and accessible biological datasets [1, 2]. These "big data" are being explored to systematically uncover useful signals and gain more insights to advance current knowledge and answer specific biological and health questions. Considering current data delude and relatively increased computing power, it is becoming possible to accurately infer desirable features from such data. This highlights the need for efficient learning algorithms to process these data for knowledge discovery by identifying pertinent patterns related to the comparison and classification of different features in these datasets. These learning algorithms should enable the extraction of appropriate features for application in a novel event or situation to support decision-making by mapping a given system to an input-output transformation task as shown in **Figure 1**. Emerging trends in (deep) machine learning algorithms have made possible the identification and discovery of new patterns and hidden processes in genomic sequences that are essential in the functioning of biological systems. The heterogeneity of diseases, such as cancer, requires primarily the analysis of genomic data in order to improve diagnosis and to design an optimal therapy for an efficient clinical management of the disease. There is an increasing need of machine learning techniques in genomic medicine.

Machine learning algorithms can be classified into three main categories, namely *supervised*, *unsupervised* and *reinforcement* learning, described below:

Supervised learning algorithms build a mapping function, f, from the input variable, X, to the output result, Y, expressed by: Y = f(X). There exist two main groups of supervised learning algorithms, namely classification and regression. Classification model is used to predict the outcome of a given sample with categorical output, for instance, case or sick individuals, labeled 0, and control or healthy individuals, labeled 1. On the other hand, a regression model is used to predict the outcome of a given sample with a real-valued output. Examples of supervised learning algorithms include logistic and linear regression models, Naive Bayes, classification and regression trees (CART) [3], K-nearest neighbor (KNN) [4, 5], support vector machine (SVM) [6], random forest (RF) [7], and artificial neural networks (ANNs) [8].

Unsupervised learning algorithms retrieve the underlying structure of the dataset based on input X only, using unlabeled data, that is, input data with no corresponding output. In this type of learning algorithm, we have: *clustering*, *dimensionality reduction*, and *association* models. Clustering consists of grouping samples so that items within the same cluster are more similar to each other than to items from another cluster for a given well-defined metric. Dimensionality reduction uses feature extraction and selection methods to reduce the number of input variables, conveying the most important information and minimizing noise in the dataset. Feature selection extracts a subset of useful variables among the original variables and transforms data from a high- to a low-dimensional space. Finally, association model just computes the probability of the co-occurrence of elements in

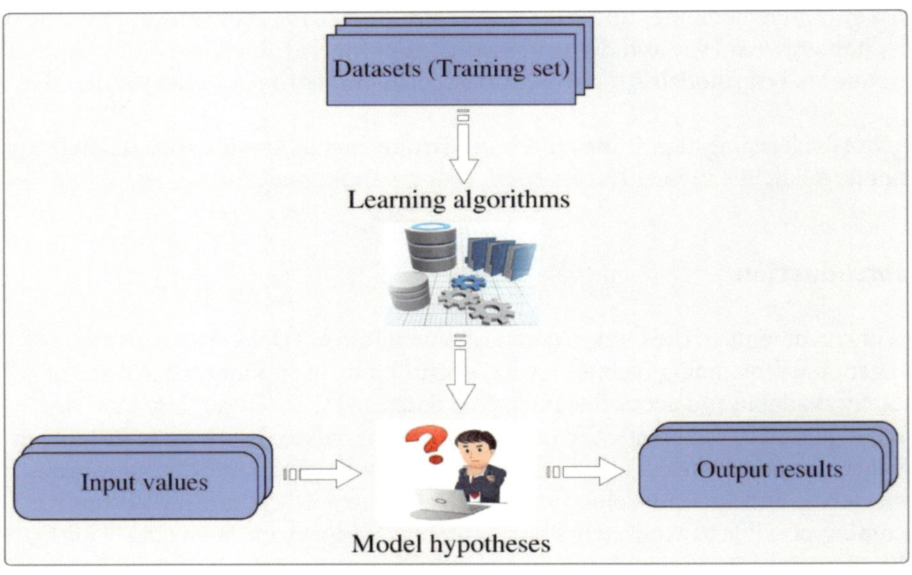

Figure 1.
Mapping a system to an input-output transformation task through learning algorithms namely supervised, unsupervised, and reinforcement learning.

a collection, thus inferring how likely two different elements are to co-occur in a collection. Unsupervised learning includes hierarchical clustering [9], K-means [10], and principal component analysis (PCA).

Reinforcement learning algorithms are a class of learning algorithms allowing an agent to decide the optimal next action based on its current state to control an environment or a system [11], by learning behaviors that will maximize the reward or outcome [12, 13]. These algorithms interact with a system, for example human system under a specific condition which may be disease or treatment, to learn the best setting and optimally perform sequential decisions along a timeline [11], generally under uncertainty, based solely on the present state of the system. It follows that this sequential and dynamic decision-making process is assumed to be a Markov decision process [14], in which the present state of the system fully describes the system and is sufficient to optimally predict the best next state. Reinforcement learning algorithms generally use a dynamic programming method following Bellman-based optimality principle [12], which requires optimal substructure for a given optimal option. In clinical research, these algorithms can be effective for longitudinal analyses, including retrospective and prospective studies, which consist of following a cohort across a specific-time interval [15].

Most of these learning algorithms have been extensively used to overcome several issues in genomic medicine, including identification of genetic markers underlying disease risk, novel mechanisms for disease prevention, control, diagnosis and therapy, building predictive disease models, predicting treatment outcomes, etc. Currently, there exist several platforms producing large-scale datasets, including genomics, transcriptomics, proteomics, metabolomics, and microbial and epidemiological data. This provides a unique opportunity of setting models and learning algorithms to enable the integration of these different heterogeneous datasets for elucidating determinant factors contributing to disease outcome and therapy in order to take full advantage of this data wealth in post-genomic medicine. In the following sections, we review some cases where machine and deep learning techniques have been used in health era and how post-genomic analysis constitutes a necessary route for optimally elucidating mechanisms of disease for an appropriate disease clinical management, and for predicting effective therapeutic strategies.

2. Use of machine learning in biology and health domains

As pointed out previously, machine learning algorithms have been successfully applied in many areas of biology and health-related research, including the identification of previously unknown processes in the genome, identification and understanding of several differentially expressed genes, binding specificities, and alternative splicing effects on cell processes, gene-gene and gene-environment interactions, disease-causing mutations, genetic determinants of diseases, pathway analysis, network and co-expression analysis, prediction of new drug-targets and response to treatment, etc. Here, we provide some illustrations of the use of supervised classification machine learning algorithms such as regression, SVM, ANN, and RF in some specific genomic applications, including predicting sequence specificities, analyzing gene expression profiles, identifying gene-gene and protein-protein interactions, and elucidating disease-associated variants.

2.1 Predicting sequence specificities of DNA- and RNA-binding proteins

Sequence specificities of DNA- and RNA-binding proteins are essential for developing models of regulatory processes in biological systems. Alipanahi et al. [16] present the possibility of predicting sequence specificities from experimental data through deep learning. They developed a software tool (DeepBind) based on deep convolutional neural networks that has the ability to discover new patterns in a sequence without knowledge of the particular location of the pattern within the sequence. DeepBind is also said to have the ability to: learn from very large amounts of sequence data through parallel implementation on a graphics processing unit (GPU); use both microarray and sequencing data; automatically train predictive models without requiring hand-tuning; tolerate mislabeled data and some noise; and generalize well across technologies regardless of existing biases across technologies. Furthermore, DeepBind was also used for identifying RNA- and DNA-binding protein sequence specificities, and showed resilience to outliers and array biases. This suggests that the issue of predicting sequence specificities has been efficiently addressed using the deep learning approach.

2.2 Analyzing gene expression profiles

With the increased availability of genome-wide gene expression assays in public databases, there is increasing demand for more efficient computational models for data interpretation. The use of artificial neural networks in biomedical research is currently taking precedence over traditional analysis methods, as they have been proven to be better classifiers. Deep neural networks, using data from RNA-seq as inputs, are being used for prediction modeling. Classic models in applications like predicting patient outcomes using gene expression data are still not effective to the expected level, thus creating a need for more efficient robust algorithms. Recent studies that use deep learning models on gene expression data have indicated better performance. Urda et al. [17] illustrated the use of a multi-layer feed-forward artificial neural network, shown in **Figure 2**, in analyzing the RNA-seq gene expression data.

Dincer et al. [18] present a model that uses variational auto-encoders (VAEs) to extract latent variables from publicly available expression datasets and use them as features for predicting phenotypes. Their system, called DeepProfile, uses deep learning to learn a feature representation from large unlabeled expression data samples that are not incorporated in the prediction problem. This system was successfully used for the prediction of response to cancer drugs based on gene expression data. It also helped determine the effects of given drugs on specific patients

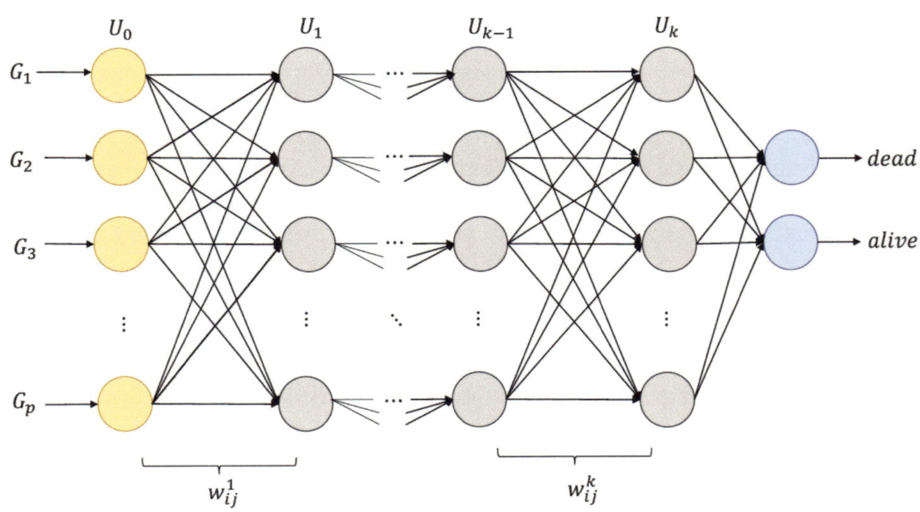

Figure 2.
Example neural network for binary classification. Input layer of P gene expression levels connected to k-hidden layers through synaptic weights w.

and thus provides a tool for precision medicine. The model was trained on gene expression data of acute myeloid leukemia, from GEO. Results indicated that low-dimensional representation (latent variables) generated using VAEs significantly outperformed the original input feature representation (gene expression levels) in the drug response prediction problem. Therefore, variational auto-encoders were shown to be effective in extracting a low-dimensional feature representation from unlabeled gene expression datasets and these learned features were found to capture important processes relevant to the prediction problem.

It is worth noting that detecting certain differentially expressed genes (DEGs) from RNA-seq results still faces challenges despite the quality control measures applied during sample preparation and data analysis. Data processing methods can lead to a certain number of false-positives and false-negatives that affect the accuracy and sensitivity of DEGs analysis. The combination of machine learning techniques with RNA-seq has been shown to significantly improve the sensitivity of DEGs [18] and thus help increase the identification of DEGs that are missed by traditional RNA-seq techniques. The study by Wang et al. [19] used a differential network analysis, based on machine learning, to predict stress-responsive genes by learning the patterns of 32 expression characteristics of known stress-related genes. For analysis using machine learning, the WEKA 3 data mining software was used for feature selection, classifier training, and evaluation. Three feature selection algorithms, correlation feature selection (CFS), information gain (InfoGain), and RELIEF [20], were used to identify features and five classifiers, logistic regression, random forest, LMT, classification via regression, and random subspace, that exhibited better performance than other machine learning algorithms, were deployed to predict up- and down-regulated genes. With this approach, the authors were able to identify the top 23 most informative features.

2.3 Inferring protein-protein interaction and biological networks for knowledge discovery

In the context of this chapter, we only focus on protein-protein interaction (PPI) network, which is defined as a set of nodes (or vertices), representing proteins connected by undirected edges (or links), which are the interactions or relationships between them (either *direct physical* or *functional* interactions). A physical interaction is an interaction that involves physical contact between proteins, and on the other hand, functional interaction, which is broad, does not necessarily involve direct physical contact, but rather refers to a mechanism through which a protein participates in cell functions [21]. Several learning algorithms have been used to infer human and human-pathogen PPIs [22], including ANN [23].

There exist several types of PPI networks based on the type of interactions and when integrated in a single network, the relationships between proteins in a unified network are referred to as functional interactions. Here, we only refer to functional interactions, which include physical and genetic interactions, and those inferred from knowledge about co-expression and shared evolutionary history or biological pathways. Other types of biological networks include signaling networks, gene regulatory or DNA-protein interaction networks [24, 25], disease-gene networks linking diseases to genes causing the disease, and drug interaction networks connecting drugs to their targets [26]. These biological networks have been used in several applications and analyzing individual, collective, and sub-network behaviors of these biological networks has enabled effective knowledge discovery at different levels of biology.

2.4 Predicting gene-gene and gene-environment interactions

Generally, disease outcome involves multiple genes contributing in every stage of disease progression [27]. This suggests the influence of gene-gene and gene-environment interactions in the outcome of a disease. Genes interact in large networks and some genes in the network are more important or central than others. Understanding these interactions is necessary for setting optimal prevention and control mechanisms to contain the disease. There have been challenges in identifying the distinctive nature of gene-gene and gene-environment interactions and their impact on disease risk, using traditional statistical methods. This has been due to the high dimensionality of the data, presence of epistasis and multiple polymorphisms leading to complex datasets for analysis. Machine learning methods such as SVM, ANN, and RF are used in addressing these challenges.

Neural networks use pattern recognition to address challenges in genomics. In the context of predicting gene-gene interaction, the neural network architecture depends on the type of interactions [28], shown in **Figure 3**. Genetic programming has been utilized to optimize the architecture of neural networks and back propagation for modeling gene-gene interactions as illustrated by Ritchie et al. [29]. Genetic programing neural nets (GPNN) were found to have more prediction power for models with heritability greater than 0.026 as compared to back propagation neural nets (BPNNs) which had only 80% power for models with greater than 0.051 heritability. The GPNN also outperformed the BPNN when applied to models containing functional and nonfunctional SNPs. Complex nonlinear interactions with binary endpoints that have previously been analyzed by logistic regression and classification and regression trees (CARTs) can be examined by GPNN. Motsinger et al. [30] demonstrated the use of grammatical evolution neural networks (GENNs) in detecting gene-gene and gene-environment interactions in high dimensional data with noise. GENN were found to be more vigorous with missing data and genotyping errors.

On the other hand, random forest (RF) algorithm is a flexible supervised machine learning algorithm that can be used for classification and regression. The RF algorithm is often able to produce good results even with missing values in the data and without need for hyper-parameter tuning. Therefore, RF algorithm can be well suited for high-dimensional genomic data analysis. This algorithm is also useful in reducing the search space of epistatic interactions, thereby creating a manageable set of possible combinations of genetic variants.

Finally, support vector machine (SVM) is a machine learning algorithm that uses hyper-planes for classification and regression tasks. The SVM approach has been applied to detecting gene-gene interactions through learning from the features of genetically interacting pairs. For training, SVM takes in two sets of feature vectors

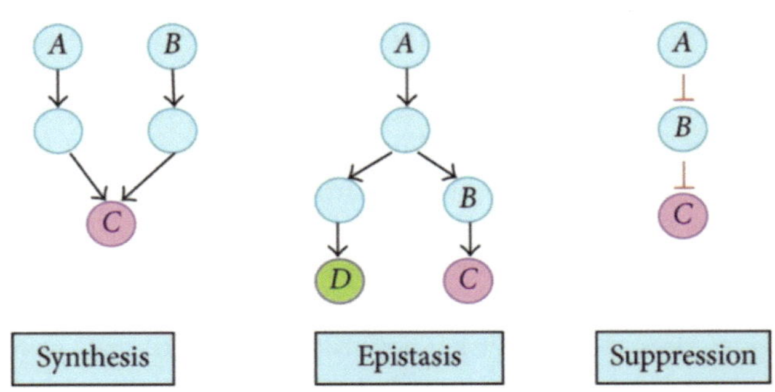

Figure 3.
Categories of gene-gene interactions retrieved from Koo et al. [23].

labeled as positive and negative, indicating presence and absence of genetic interaction, respectively. Feature mapping is done by use of a hyper-plane with maximum margin to separate genetically interacting pairs and non-genetically interacting pairs. SVM and neural network modeling was used to investigate gene-gene interactions in a study by Matchenko-Shimko and Dube [31]. They used pre-selection of SNP-SNP combination to determine the effects of interactions between genes. However, the pre-selection strategy did not work well with combinations of low disease allele frequencies and low margin effects. It was discovered that larger sample sizes are required for determining gene-gene interactions with SNPs having low marginal effect sizes as compared to interactions with moderate marginal gene effect sizes. Both SVM and ANN models exhibited good performance in increasing allele frequency with low marginal gene effects [31]. SVM was used to identify the most promising SNPs and interactions. Shen et al. used it in two stages for determining gene-gene interactions where the second stage involves the application of logistic regression analysis. It was shown that SVM is also useful in methods for case-control studies in which multiple logistic regression performs better than traditional logistic regression for each interaction. Additionally, application of the SVM in improving the accuracy of cancer classification, through extending the SVM pedigree-based generalized multifactor dimensionality, has been functional in detecting gene-gene and gene-covariate interactions in limited family samples [32]. Moreover, the SVM can also be used to extract known gene-disease associations and infer known genes for future experimental analysis using automatic literature mining based on dependency parsing and SVM [33].

In addition, the application of SVM in SUPPORTMIX [34], which is a local ancestry inference method, facilitates gene-gene and gene-environment interactions. For instance, Aschard et al. [35] highlighted that local ancestry estimates might provide insights into detecting gene-gene interactions, while Florez et al. [36] showed that non-European ancestry in the Latino populations is associated with type 2 diabetes and lower economic status, illustrating gene-environment interaction. Local ancestry inference estimates the proportion of alleles that originates from a particular population at every chromosomal site of an admixed individual. SUPPORTMIX integrates SVM with hidden Markov models (HMMs). Using SVM in SUPPORTMIX improves multi-way local ancestry inference overall, since it addresses the challenge of few genotyped or existing reference panels [1]. Furthermore, it facilitates both gene-gene and gene-environment interactions due to the improved computational time as a result of its flexibility and ability to handle "big data."

2.5 Elucidating disease-causing genetic variants

The identification of disease-causing genetic variants is challenging because several of them are found in the non-coding regions of the genome. The role of non-coding regions in the maintenance of genome functions is not well understood. However, some machine learning algorithms have been designed to annotate coding and non-coding genetic variants in order to identify disease-causing mutations. *Combined annotation-dependent depletion* (CADD) is an algorithm designed to annotate coding and non-coding variants [37]. CADD trains a linear kernel support vector machine to separate observed genetic variants from simulated ones. However, due to the SVM's inability to capture nonlinear relationships among features, a deep neural network that uses the same feature set and training data as CADD is preferred. Deep neural networks are better suited than SVMs for problems with large samples and features.

How genetic variants, especially those which are not within protein coding regions, affect RNA splicing is not entirely understood. This type of problem can however be addressed by machine learning computational models designed to predict splicing during gene expression. Regulation of splicing is very important and faulty regulation could lead to several diseases, such as cancer and neurological disorders. A computational technique, that scores the magnitude of the effects of genetic variants on RNA splicing, was developed by Xiong et al. [38]. The computational model can be applied to any sequence with a triplet of exons and used to determine how splicing is altered by genetic variants. The model computes a score that predicts how much a given variant affects splicing.

Linkage and *association analysis* are types of neural network methods used to identify genes associated with diseases. Linkage analysis is used to detect the connection between a disease locus and a marker and uses genotypes as inputs and the outputs are phenotype values such as disease status and quantitative clinical variables. Association analysis on the other hand is used for detecting the disequilibrium between disease locus and marker. The data in association analysis are of case-control type with a sample comprised of genotypes for multiple markers. In most cases, it is useful to integrate genotype information into pathway analysis for more effective biological interpretation of these genotype contributions into the trait under consideration. In this case, *random survival forest pathway hunting* algorithm can be used to identify signaling pathways in a relatively small sample size [39].

Finally, considering the RF features, the RF algorithm can also be used in identifying a set of risk-associated SNPs from a large number of unassociated SNPs in models of complex diseases. There are unknown interactions among true risk-associated SNPs or SNPs and the environment in large-scale genetic data and RF can be used to significantly reduce the number of SNPs in the data as pointed out previously.

2.6 Applying learning algorithms in clinical decision process

Setting appropriate diagnostic and effective therapeutic regimens is a critical clinical decision and essential for setting effective health measures and efficient strategies to control a disease. This process is limited by the lack of advanced diagnostic tools and approved therapy or vaccine against most existing and emerging diseases [40, 41]. Moreover, despite undeniable advances made in understanding of human biology, etiology, and pathogenesis of several diseases, and emergence of advanced technologies, the translation of the existing biological knowledge toward effective new treatments and clinical interventions has not been as fast as expected or anticipated. This highlights the need for powerful and general tools for orienting these clinical decision processes. Machine learning algorithms are contributing to satisfying this need with several advantages in representational power even though challenges in biological interpretation still hamper clinical applications [15].

As an initial illustration, Adabor and Acquaah-Mensah [42] introduced the median supplement model to appropriately balance a training set with unequal numbers of instances associated with each class or group to improve the classification decision. They also assessed different machine learning techniques in predicting the receptor expression status of breast cancer patients, namely progesterone receptor (PR) status and HER2 expression status using gene expression datasets. These receptors are essential in deciding on treatment and predicting the treatment outcome. In this chapter, we used results of their performance evaluations to highlight two essential features common to most of the machine learning algorithms as shown in **Figure 4**: (1) as the size of the training set increases, the performance of the learning algorithm increases (see Sample Data 1 vs. Sample Data 2) and (2) learning algorithm on a balanced training set may perform better than on an unbalanced training set (see NB vs. MNB and RF vs. MRF).

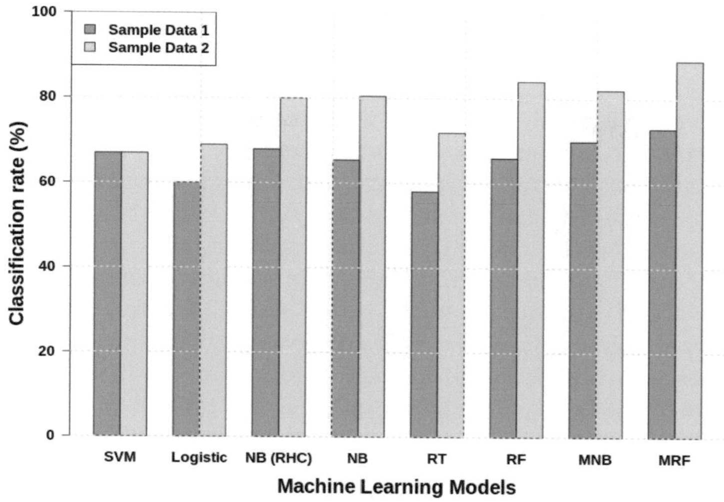

Figure 4.
Performance of different machine learning techniques for predicting progesterone receptor (PR) status phenotype of breast cancer patients based on classification rate (proportion of correctly classified instances), information extracted from [42]. Sample Data 1 is a smaller-sized dataset as compared to sample data 2, containing 162 and 1146 instances of breast cancer patients, respectively. Learning techniques: support vector machine (SVM), logistic regression (logistic), Bayesian network (BN), Naive Bayes (NB), random trees (RT), random forest (RF), median-supplement Naive Bayes (MNB), and median-supplement random forest (MRF).

It is worth mentioning that machine learning algorithms have been used in several contexts with a common goal of improving healthcare measures and patient clinical management. For examples, deep learning algorithms are used to classify patients based on clinical healthcare records [43], to predict the effectiveness of clinical trials (i.e., likelihood of success or failure of clinical trials) [44], to improve and predict patient treatment response and outcome based on pharmaco-genomics data [45]. Moreover, Nemati et al. [14] optimized a treatment dosing policy for intensive care patients using deep reinforcement learning and Wang et al. [46] predicted drug-target binding site interactions using ANN with two hidden layers taking a drug and a target binding site as inputs. Finally, it is known that drug repositioning or re-purposing approach, which examines new therapeutic uses for approved drugs, represents an optimal model for suggesting new drugs using drug-target interactions [40, 41]. Wang and Zeng [47] used a learning technique based on restricted Boltzmann machines to predict novel drug-target interactions directing to drug re-purposing.

3. Integrative approaches for post-genomic analysis

Over the years, thousands of genetic associations have been discovered using genetic approach, known as *genome-wide association studies* (GWAS). GWAS approaches are mostly based on a single-marker association test model that leverages thousands of genomes of cases and controls (sick and healthy individuals) in order to elucidate variants or single-nucleotide polymorphisms (SNPs) with unusual significant differences in frequency throughout genomes [48]. This indicates that GWAS approaches are based on machine learning techniques, which mostly take SNP profiles of cases and controls as inputs, and predict a SNP carrying disease risk. Note that these approaches have been successful [49] and several GWAS results have helped elucidating genetic determinants of susceptibility to several diseases, including complex diseases, such as cancer, and monogenic diseases, such as sickle cell disease. In fact, in case of the breast cancer disease, a genetic testing tool has been implemented [50] based on specific genetic variants in breast cancer type 1 (BRCA1) and 2 (BRCA2) susceptibility genes in chromosomes 17 (17q21.31) and 13 (13q13.1) [51], respectively. It is widely known that the outcome of a disease, in particular a complex disease, or a response to a drug is influenced by multiple genes and significant contribution from the environment. This strongly argues that using only genomic analysis will not be sufficient to entirely embed phenotypic variation and heritability, suggesting that genomic analysis alone is not sufficient to elucidate the complex structure of the disease [52]. Thus, there is a significant need of integrating information derived from environmental studies and other heterogeneous datasets into genomic analysis to enhance the predictive power of genomic analysis.

As indicated above, even though genomic information is critical, it is not sufficient to completely elucidate disease outcome and progression, which involve gene-gene and gene-environment interactions. In this context, the post-genomic analysis may provide a new paradigm to genomic analysis and may enable further functional characterization of genetic susceptibility to a disease and correlate disease-associated (candidate) genes by combining association signals from genomic analysis and available knowledge, including functional, environmental, epidemiological, and clinical information. This integrative approach increases the likelihood of effectively identifying suitable candidate genes [53] and biological pathways that may be critical in the etiology and pathogenesis of the disease, and in the drug response. The next goal is to integrate large-scale datasets from heterogeneous sources [2, 54] to move beyond a single genomic approach and foster a whole genome-based integrative approach to achieve global view [55]. A biological network, which is a network modeling a biological system as an entity composed of sub-units connected as a whole, has become a useful tool enabling the integration of heterogeneous datasets into a single framework [26].

4. Challenges and perspectives

Currently, there is an exponential growth of several platforms producing large-scale datasets, including genomics, transcriptomics, proteomics, metabolomics, microbial and epidemiological data. These high-dimensional datasets from heterogeneous sources create an opportunity of designing appropriate data-driven learning algorithms and models to ensure effective post-genomic medicine and biomedical research with an increased prediction power. While the use of these large-scale post-genomic datasets from heterogeneous sources, such as transcriptomics, proteomics, metabolomics, microbial and epidemiological data, shows several potential advantages and opportunities, many challenges still exist in terms of computational models, learning algorithms, and biological interpretation of result outputs. Furthermore, as discussed previously, learning, reinforcement, and deep learning algorithms are quickly evolving with several potential applications in biology and medicine (see **Section 2.6**). Currently, predictions from different models are unable to contribute to clinical decision processes as the effectiveness of these models still poses problems in the absence of ground-truth, gold standard (benchmark) datasets, or experimental validation. This suggests that one of the future trend aspects of learning algorithms in biology and medicine will be to make possible the integration of predictive models generated by these learning algorithms into dynamic clinical settings. This integration will necessitate that issues raised above are addressed systematically and will ensure an effective exploitation of the post-genomic datasets and potentially revolutionize the study of human disease and health.

Machine intelligence and deep learning models present more powerful computational techniques that are able to effectively learn from large complex datasets in order to reveal several hidden interactions within cell variables and give more insight into the intricate processes linked to diseases [56]. On the other hand, despite the current undoubted data wealth, we still have a very limited understanding of the mechanisms underlying the outcome, pathogenesis, and progress of many diseases, which is reflected in an existing gap between this data wealth and translation toward enhancing treatment and interventions for diseases, leading to the paradigm of "world with data wealth and information poor". This is partly due to issues related to different existing datasets, including: (1) increased heterogeneity within a dataset as, in general, these datasets are collected across different locations, thus lacking a standardized representation of the data and (2) variation of cohorts in terms of size across populations and geographical locations. This highlights the need for designing adequate meta-analysis models to assist in retrieving useful information within each data source. This may also require more advanced machine learning techniques to play an important role in genomic medicine and advance our knowledge about disease and health.

5. Conclusions

Numerous large-scale platforms have been designed for producing different types of high-dimensional datasets, including genomics, transcriptomics, proteomics, metabolomics, microbial and epidemiological data. This data deluge provides a rich source of information, which can advance our understanding of human and pathogenic organisms to enhance post-genomic medicine and biomedical research. In this chapter, we have provided some illustrations of machine learning algorithms for knowledge discovery in biological and health areas and discussed existing challenges. This discussion highlights the need for adequate meta-analysis-based post-genomic models to optimally integrate diverse datasets from different sources. This clearly suggests that initial machine learning algorithms will need to be refined or new ones need to be developed to account for current data challenges in order to speed up the translation of the current and future knowledge into effective new treatment strategies and health measures, enabling efficient clinical disease management and ensuring effective post-genomic medicine.

Conflict of interest

The authors declare that they have no competing interests.

Author details

Gaston K. Mazandu[1,2,3*], Irene Kyomugisha[2,4], Ephifania Geza[2,3], Milaine Seuneu[2], Bubacarr Bah[2,4] and Emile R. Chimusa[1]

1 Division of Human Genetics, Department of Pathology, Institute of Infectious Disease and Molecular Medicine, Faculty of Health Sciences, University of Cape Town (UCT), Cape Town, South Africa

2 African Institute for Mathematical Sciences (AIMS), Cape Town, South Africa

3 Computational Biology (CBIO) Division, Department of Integrative Biomedical Science, Institute of Infectious Disease and Molecular Medicine, Faculty of Health Sciences, University of Cape Town (UCT), Cape Town, South Africa

4 Division of Applied Mathematics, Department of Mathematical Sciences, University of Stellenbosch, Stellenbosch, South Africa

*Address all correspondence to: kuzamunu@aims.ac.za

References

[1] Geza E, Mugo J, Mulder NJ, Wonkam A, Chimusa ER, Mazandu GK. A comprehensive survey of models for dissecting local ancestry deconvolution in human genome. Briefings in Bioinformatics. 2018:1-16

[2] Mazandu GK, Chimusa ER, Mulder NJ. Gene ontology semantic similarity tools: Survey on features and challenges for biological knowledge discovery. Briefings in Bioinformatics. 2016;**18**(5):886-901

[3] Strobl C, Malley J, Gerhard T. Characteristics of classification and regression trees, bagging and random forests. Psychological Methods. 2009;**14**(4):323-348

[4] Altman NS. An introduction to kernel and nearest-neighbor nonparametric regression. The American Statistician. 1992;**46**(3):175-185

[5] Khondoker M, Dobson R, Skirrow C, Simmons A, Stahl D. A comparison of machine learning methods for classification using simulation with multiple real data examples from mental health studies. Statistical Methods in Medical Research. 2016;**25**(5):1804-1823

[6] Cortes C, Vapnik V. Support-vector networks. Machine Learning. 1995;**20**(3):273-297

[7] Breiman L. Random forests. Machine Learning. 2001;**45**(1):5-32

[8] Karpathy A. CS231n Convolutional Neural Networks for Visual Recognition. Available from: http://cs231n.github.io/neural-networks-1/#nn 2017

[9] Murtagh F, Contreras P. Algorithms for hierarchical clustering: An overview. Wiley Interdisciplinary Reviews: Data Mining and Knowledge Discovery. 2012;2:86-97. 7 (2017) e1219

[10] Hartigan JA, Wong MA. Algorithm AS 136: A k-means clustering algorithm. Journal of the Royal Statistical Society, Series C. 1979;**28**(1):100-108

[11] Bothe MK, Dickens L, Reichel K, Tellmann A, Ellger B, Westphal M, et al. The use of reinforcement learning algorithms to meet the challenges of an artificial pancreas. Expert Review of Medical Devices. 2013;**10**(5):661-673

[12] Weng WH, Gao M, He Z, Yan S, Szolovits P. Representation and reinforcement learning for personalized glycemic control in septic patients. In: 31st Conference on Neural Information Processing Systems (NIPS); Long Beach, CA, USA. 2017

[13] Ling Y, Hasan SA, Datla V, Qadir A, Lee K, Liu J, et al. Learning to diagnose: assimilating clinical narratives using deep reinforcement learning. In: Proceedings of the 8th International Joint Conference on Natural Language Processing. 2017. pp. 895-905

[14] Nemati S, Ghassemi MM, Clifford GD. Optimal medication dosing from suboptimal clinical examples: A deep reinforcement learning approach. In: Conference Proceedings: Annual International Conference of the IEEE Engineering in Medicine and Biology Society. 2016. pp. 2978-2981. DOI: 10.1109/EMBC.2016.7591355

[15] Ching T, Himmelstein DS, Beaulieu-Jones BK, Kalinin AA, Do BT, et al. Opportunities and obstacles for deep learning in biology and medicine. Journal of the Royal Society Interface. 2018;**15**. DOI: 10.1098/rsif.2017.0387

[16] Alipanahi B, Delong A, Weirauch MT, Frey BJ. Predicting the sequence specificities of DNA- and RNA-binding proteins by deep learning. Nature Biotechnology. 2015;**33**(8):831-838

[17] Urda D, Montes-Torres J, Moreno F, Franco L, Jerez JM. Deep learning to analyze RNA-seq gene expression data. In: International Work-Conference on Artificial Neural Networks. Springer; 2017. pp. 50-59

[18] Dincer AB, Celik S, Hiranuma N, Lee S. DeepProfile: Deep learning of cancer molecular profiles for precision medicine. bioRxiv 2018. 278739. DOI: 10.1101/278739

[19] Wang L, Xi Y, Sung S, Qiao H. RNA-seq assistant: machine learning based methods to identify more transcriptional regulated genes. BMC Genomics. 2018;**19**:546

[20] Rosario SF, Thangadurai K. RELIEF: Feature selection approach. International Journal of Innovation Science and Research. 2015;**4**(11):218-224

[21] Mazandu GK, Mulder NJ. Generation and analysis of large-scale data-driven Mycobacterium tuberculosis functional networks for drug target identification. Advances in Bioinformatics. 2011;**2011**:801478

[22] Rapanoel HA, Mazandu GK, Mulder NJ. Predicting and analyzing interactions between Mycobacterium tuberculosis and its human host. PLoS One. 2013;**8**(7):e67472

[23] Ahmed I, Witbooi P, Christoffels A. Prediction of human-*Bacillus anthracis* protein-protein interactions using multi-layer neural network. Bioinformatics. 2018;**34**(24):4159-4164

[24] Pavlopoulos GA, Secrier M, Moschopoulos CN, Soldatos TG, Kossida S, Aerts J, et al. Using graph theory to analyze biological networks. BioData Mining. 2011;**4**:10

[25] Alm E, Arkin PA. Biological networks. Current Opinion in Structural Biology. 2013;**13**:193-202

[26] Ma'ayan A. Introduction to Network Analysis in Systems Biology. Science Signaling. 2011;**4**(190):tr5

[27] Mazandu GK, Mulder NJ. Enhancing drug target identification in Mycobacterium tuberculosis. In: Tuberculosis: Risk Factors, Drug Resistance and Treatment. NOVA Publishers; 2012

[28] Koo CL, Liew MJ, Mohamad MS, Salleh AHM. A review for detecting gene-gene interactions using machine learning methods in genetic epidemiology. BioMed Research International. 2013;**2013**:432375

[29] Ritchie MD, White BC, Parker JS, Hahn LW, Moore JH. Optimization of neural network architecture using genetic programming improves detection and modelling of gene-gene interactions in studies of human diseases. BMC Bioinformatics. 2003;**4**:28

[30] Motsinger-Reif AA, Fanelli TJ, Davis AC, Ritchie MD. Power of grammatical evolution neural networks to detect gene-gene interactions in the presence of error. BMC Research Notes. 2008;**1**:65

[31] Matchenko-Shimko N, Dube MP. Gene-gene interaction tests using SVM and neural network modeling. In: 2007 Proceedings of the IEEE Symposium on Computational Intelligence in Bioinformatics and Computational Biology. 2006. pp. 90-97

[32] Fang Y, Chiu Y. SVM-based generalized multifactor dimensionality reduction approaches for detecting gene-gene interactions in family studies. Genetic Epidemiology. 2012;**36**(2):88-98

[33] Ozgur A, Vu T, Erkan G, Radev DR. Identifying gene-disease associations using centrality on a literature mined gene-interaction network. Bioinformatics. 2008;**24**(13):i277-i285

[34] Omberg L, Salit J, Hackett N, Fuller J, Matthew R, Chouchane L, et al. Inferring genome-wide patterns of admixture in Qataris using fifty-five ancestral populations. BMC Genetics. 2012, 2012;**13**(1):49

[35] Aschard H, Gusev A, Brown R, Pasaniuc B. Leveraging local ancestry to detect gene-gene interactions in genome-wide data. BMC Genetics. 2015;**16**:124

[36] Florez JC, Price AL, Campbell D, Riba L, Parra MV, Yu F, et al. Strong association of socioeconomic status with genetic ancestry in Latinos: Implications for admixture studies of type 2 diabetes. Diabetologia. 2009;**52**(8):1528-1536

[37] Quang D, Chen Y, Xie X. DANN: A deep learning approach for annotating the pathogenicity of genetic variants. Bioinformatics. 2014;**31**(5):761-763

[38] Xiong HY, Alipanahi B, Lee LJ, Bretschneider H, Merico D, Yuen RKC, et al. The human splicing code reveals new insights into the genetic determinants of disease. Science. 2015;**347**(6218):1254806

[39] Chen X, Ishwaran H. Pathway hunting by random forests. Bioinformatics. 2013;**29**(1):99-105

[40] Mazandu GK, Chimusa ER, Rutherford K, Zekeng EG, Gebremariam ZZ, Onifade MY, et al. Large-scale data-driven integrative framework for extracting essential targets and processes from disease-associated gene data sets. Briefings in Bioinformatics. 2018;**19**(6):1141-1152. DOI: 10.1093/bib/bbx052

[41] Rutherford KD, Mazandu GK, Mulder NJ. A systems-level analysis of drug-target-disease associations for drug repositioning. Briefings in Functional Genomics. 2017;**17**(1):34-41

[42] Adabor ES, Acquaah-Mensah GK. Machine learning approaches to decipher hormone and HER2 receptor status phenotypes in breast cancer. Briefings in Bioinformatics. 2017. DOI: 10.1093/bib/bbx138

[43] Huddar V, Desiraju BK, Rajan V, Bhattacharya S, Roy S, Reddy CK. Predicting complications in critical care using heterogeneous clinical data. IEEE Access. 2016;**4**:7988-8001. DOI: 10.1109/access.2016.2618775

[44] Artemov AV, Putin E, Vanhaelen Q, Aliper A, Ozerov IV, Zhavoronkov A. Integrated deep learned transcriptomic and structure-based predictor of clinical trials outcomes. bioRxiv. 2016. doi: 10.1101/095653

[45] Kalinin AA, Higgins GA, Reamaroon N, Reza SM, Allyn-Feuer A, Dinov ID, Najarian K, Athey BD. Deep learning in pharmacogenomics: From gene regulation to patient stratification. 2018. https://arxiv.org/abs/1801.08570v1

[46] Wang C, Liu J, Luo F, Tan Y, Deng Z, Hu QN. Pairwise input neural network for target-ligand interaction prediction. In: 2014 IEEE International Conference on BIBM. 2014. pp. 67-70

[47] Wang Y, Zeng J. Predicting drug-target interactions using restricted Boltzmann machines. Bioinformatics. 2013;**29**:i126-i134

[48] Chimusa ER, Dalvie S, Dandara C, Wonkam A, Mazandu GK. Post genome-wide association analysis: Dissecting computational pathway/network-based approaches. Briefings in Bioinformatics. DOI: 10.1093/bib/bby035

[49] Welter D, MacArthur J, Morales J, Burdett T, Hall P, Junkins H, et al. The NHGRI GWAS Catalog, a curated resource of SNP-trait associations. Nucleic Acids Research;**42**:D1001-D1006

[50] Gabai-Kapara E, Lahad A, Kaufman B, Friedman E, Segev S, Renbaum P,

et al. Population-based screening for breast and ovarian cancer risk due to BRCA1 and BRCA2. PNAS. 2014;**111**(39):14205-14210

[51] Försti A, Luo L, Vorechovsky I, Söderberg M, Lichtenstein P, Hemminki K. Allelic imbalance on chromosomes 13 and 17 and mutation analysis of BRCA1 and BRCA2 genes in monozygotic twins concordant for breast cancer. Carcinogenesis. 2001;**22**(1):27-33

[52] Chimusa ER, Mbiyavanga M, Mazandu GK, Mulder NJ. AncGWAS: A post genome-wide association study method for interaction, pathway, and ancestry analysis in homogeneous and admixed populations. Bioinformatics. 2016;**32**(4):549-556

[53] Ma X, Gao L. Biological network analysis: Insights into structure and functions. Briefings in Functional Genomics. 2012;**11**(6):434-442

[54] Mulder NJ, Akinola RO, Mazandu GK, Rapanoel H. Using biological networks to improve our understanding of infectious diseases. Computational and Structural Biotechnology Journal. 2014;**11**(18):1-10

[55] Mazandu GK, Opap K, Mulder NJ. Contribution of microarray data to the advancement of knowledge on the Mycobacterium tuberculosis interactome: Use of the random partial least squares approach. Infection, Genetics and Evolution. 2011;**11**(4):725-733

[56] Leung MKK, Xiong HY, Lee LJ, Frey BJ. Deep learning of the tissue-regulated splicing code. Bioinformatics. 2014;**30**(12):i121-i129

Chapter 2

A Review of EMG Techniques for Detection of Gait Disorders

Rajat Emanuel Singh, Kamran Iqbal, Gannon White and Jennifer K. Holtz

Abstract

Electromyography (EMG) is a commonly used technique to record myoelectric signals, i.e., motor neuron signals that originate from the central nervous system (CNS) and synergistically activate groups of muscles resulting in movement. EMG patterns underlying movement, recorded using surface or needle electrodes, can be used to detect movement and gait abnormalities. In this review article, we examine EMG signal processing techniques that have been applied for diagnosing gait disorders. These techniques span from traditional statistical tests to complex machine learning algorithms. We particularly emphasize those techniques are promising for clinical applications. This study is pertinent to both medical and engineering research communities and is potentially helpful in advancing diagnostics and designing rehabilitation devices.

Keywords: electromyography, feature extraction, classification, gait disorders, machine learning, time-frequency analysis

1. Introduction

EMG is an electrodiagnostic technique used to record the electrical activity in skeletal muscles. EMG signals are complex and exhibit intricate patterns that are dependent on the anatomical properties of the muscle [1–3]. The signal manifests the neuromuscular activation underlying muscle contraction [1, 3]. Therefore, an abnormality in the contraction of a muscle due to an injury, nerve damage, or muscular or neurological disorder that causes motor dysfunction can be identified through EMG signal diagnosis. The motor neuron signal carries information from the CNS aimed for limb displacement by flexing and extending the joints [4, 5]. The dynamic electrical activity of these motor units is called motor unit action potentials (MUAPs). These are super-positioned and recorded by the EMG device [6]. EMG can be recorded using surface electrodes, fine wire electrodes as well as anal and vaginal probes for pelvic floor muscles [2]. A simple model of an EMG signal is given by Eq. (1), where, $y(n)$ is the sampled EMG signal, $a(r)$ is the MUAP, $x(n)$ is point processed firing impulse, w_n is the white Gaussian noise and N is the number of motor unit firing at a particular time.

$$y(n) = \sum_{i=1}^{N-1} a_i(r)\, x_i(n-r) + w_n \qquad (1)$$

Our aim in this article is to review EMG signal processing techniques that facilitate detection of gait and movement disorders. We discuss techniques from simple enveloping to complex computational machine learning algorithms that may help detect alterations in EMG patterns while performing daily life activities. We may note that there are number of highly cited review articles such as Raez et al. [7], and Chowdhury et al. [8], that review EMG processing and classification techniques. The novelty in our review is that in addition to discussing innovative processing techniques we have emphasized their applications, particularly focusing on lower limb disorders. In Section 2, we review the basic techniques such as EMG enveloping, followed by EMG onset/offset detection in Section 3. In Section 4, we review current literature on the decomposition of EMG signals into MUAPs and muscle synergies. In Section 5, we discuss the analysis of the EMG signal in the frequency and time-frequency domain to understand changes due to motor impairment. When working with a larger sample size, a machine learning system can be used to classify subjects with altered muscle activation and abnormal gait patterns [9, 10]. In Section 6, we discuss algorithms that employ supervised and unsupervised learning to detect patterns of gait disorders, followed by a discussion of future trends and conclusion in Section 7.

2. EMG envelopes

Visual inspection of the raw EMG plot or its envelope requires high dexterity and clinical experience to detect motor impairment. The methodology to obtain the EMG envelope includes preprocessing, signal filtering, rectification, smoothing, standardization, statistical testing, and intricate computational algorithms. Scientific recommendations by SENIAM project and International society of electromyography and Kinesiology (ISEK) suggest use of bandpass filters (10–500 Hz) to reduce aliasing effects when using a sampling frequency of 1 kHz. Intramuscular and needle recordings should be made with the low-pass cut-off set at 1500 Hz. Avoiding notch filter is recommended as it destroys the signal information [2]. De Luca et al. recommended root mean square (RMS) value to compute the signal amplitude of the EMG during voluntary contraction [3]. Methods to form EMG envelopes include moving average, root mean square, spline interpolation over local maxima, integrated EMG etc. EMG envelope can also be obtained from low pass Butterworth 6 Hz filter. Hilbert finite impulse response (FIR) filter computes magnitude of the analytic EMG signal.

A decrease in EMG amplitude was visually observable for chronic spinal cord injury (SCI) patients while walking for 3 min [11]. Biceps femoris (BF) and gastrocnemius medial (GM) revealed consistent activity, but that was not the case for tibialis anterior (TA) and rectus femoris (RF). The RMS magnitude of the signal from BF and GM muscles decreased with longer activity duration (10 min) followed by an EMG burst resulting from muscle spasm. Identification of chronic SCI was done by simple visual inspection of the raw EMG [11]. The inter-neuronal degradation was the cause of decreased locomotor performance [11]. The RMS amplitude of the EMG signal using a paired t-test showed a higher duration of muscle activity for BF and TA among cervical spondylotic myelopathic patients (CSM) [12]. The amplitude of the muscle burst activity was not statistically different between the healthy group and CSM [12]. The muscle stretch analyzed from kinematic data did not relate with spasticity, but the ratio of EMG RMS amplitude to the mechanomyogram data showed statistically significant results for healthy and myotonic control groups [12, 13].

The stochastic and nonstationary nature of EMG signals makes it harder to study the innate patterns of the electrical activity of the muscles. Statistical tests such as Pearson's, Pearson's r, the Kolmogorov-Smirnov T-test, ANOVA F ratio and t-test, and Wilcoxon Signed Rank Test can demonstrate significant changes in the EMG profiles associated with different behavior [14, 15]. Domingo et al. performed an ANOVA on the normalized EMG amplitude of spinal cord injured patients, which led to the conclusion that with increased speed and no manual assistance the EMG pattern exhibited statistical significance when compared to the control group. The shape and timing of EMG patterns were less similar to controls [16]. Among stroke patients, the EMG activity displayed heterogeneity in comparison with healthy individuals [17]. Nieuwboer et al. [18] demonstrated that raw EMG and its linear envelopes of Parkinson's patients during freezing episodes displayed abnormal activity of TA and GM. Nonparametric tests on the RMS EMG envelope of the hemiplegic patient showed statistical significance during push off and early stance phase [14]. EMG data acquired from Parkinson patients' shoulder muscles revealed higher activation than those of healthy control subjects [19]. Average and maximum EMG amplitude were calculated for comparison [19].

Traditional statistical testing of the EMG uses ANOVA techniques that may not identify visually differentiable waveform features. McKay et al. [20] developed a more reliable statistical method to find the underlying patterns with the wavelet-based functional test (wfANOVA). Its performance to detect the changes in the magnitude and shape of EMG was more precise than the time domain ANOVA test. Wilcoxon signed rank tests were also used in studies with non-parametric data [12]. EMG envelope extraction using time domain features from multichannel sensors and their statistical tests can assist in the detection of altered myoelectric activity. Specific features such as EMG onset/offset, MUAP etc. can be analyzed from the envelopes for the diagnosis of gait disorders. **Figure 1** shows signal envelope extracted from the EMG signal with RMS. MATLAB functions were used to extract envelope and perform a statistical hypothesis test for a healthy individual and other disorders.

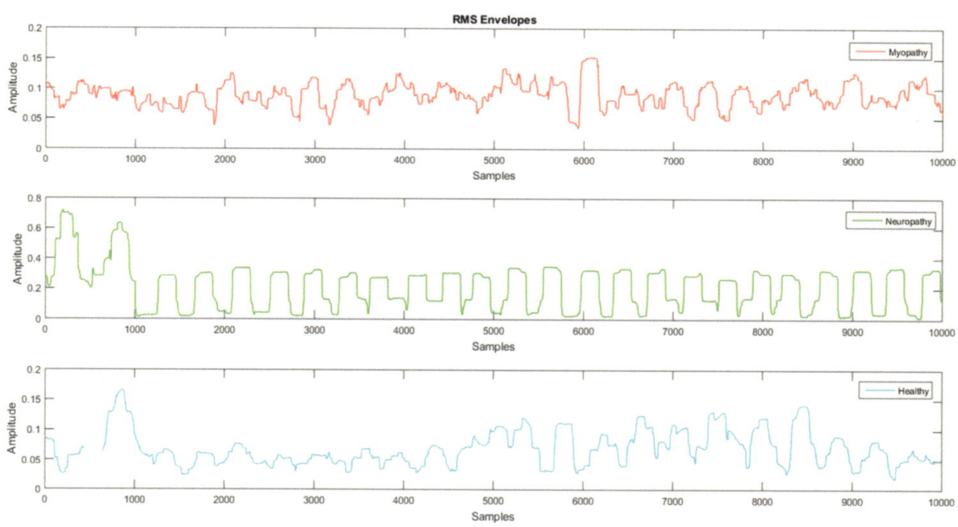

Figure 1.
RMS envelope from a healthy, a myopathic, and a neuropathic patient. A non-overlapping window of 200 samples was used and a paired student t-test revealed statistical significance ($p < 0.05$) between healthy and neuropathic, and healthy and myopathic conditions. The data was obtained from physionet [21].

3. EMG onset detection

EMG onset parameters define the duration for the muscles to stay active [2]. Onset estimation is useful to diagnose abnormality in muscle coordination. To detect the EMG onset, visual inspection or measurement of nerve conduction velocity may be used [22]. The basic thresholding method for onset detection is sensitive to the type of trials, EMG amplifiers and noise level in the signal. The thresholding based on SD baseline noise can be improved with local peak value. In a study [23], integrated EMG provided more information about early activation. During preconditioning, Teager-Kaiser Energy Operator (TKEO) also improved the onset detection accuracy by constricting the energy of the baseline noise [24, 25]. Staude et al. compared onset detection methods based on the statistical optimal decision threshold [26]. The simple threshold algorithm of Hodges and Bui [26] identifies the onset at a point where the mean of the samples within a fixed time window surpasses the baseline level by a defined multiple of standard deviation [27].

The basic framework of the threshold detection algorithm includes signal conditioning (rectification, filtering, whitening etc.), detection (Test Function and Decision rule), and postprocessing [26]. A block diagram is shown in **Figure 2**.

Double threshold methods are considered better in comparison to single threshold methods [7]. The Bonato algorithm [28] includes pre-whitening filter and data sample squaring in the conditioning unit. The test function is computed between two successive samples from the conditioned EMG signal. The onset point identification is based on the following rules: (1) x out of y samples must exceed the threshold and (2) activation state of the muscle after surpassing the threshold should last for a certain number of samples or duration of time [26].

In Lidierth [29] method, the signal conditioning unit performs full wave rectification. The test function and decision rule are based on Hodges [26]. Additional post-processing rules increase the efficiency of the algorithm. The test function unit detects the onset if the sEMG signal exceeds the threshold. Any decline in the activity below threshold within a defined duration, should not be longer than the defined range of samples [29]. The power spectral correlation coefficient method performs better than TKEO and utilizes the moving average method of Hodges and Bui [30]. The statistical estimation algorithm includes an optimal estimator and approximated generalized likelihood-ratio detector. The statistically optimized algorithms are more robust in terms of signal parameters [26]. Tenan et al. [25] reviewed three classes of standard EMG (linear envelope, entropy, TKEO) and

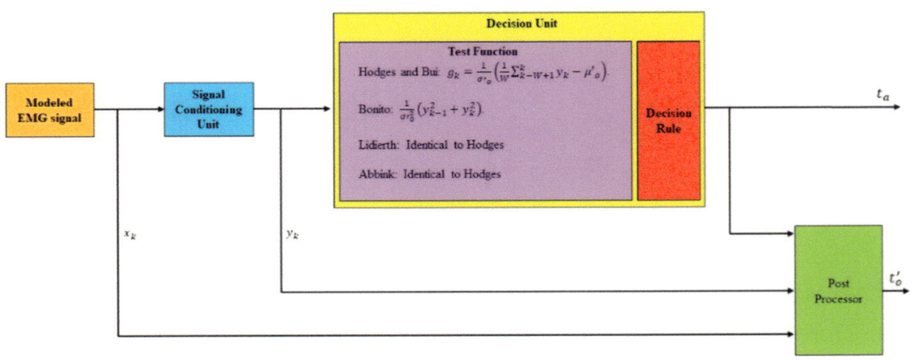

Figure 2.
EMG onset estimation framework; x_k is Gaussian noise signal, y_k is the processed signal, σ'_o and μ'_o are standard deviation and mean of samples, respectively, $g_k \geq Th$ (Threshold) is the value to trigger an alarm t_a, and t'_o is the change time estimation.

six classes of statistical EMG onset detection (general time series/mean–variance, sequential change point detection with parametric and non-parametric methods, batch change point detection, and Bayesian change point analysis). The Bayesian Change Point analysis algorithm showed higher reliability and accuracy for the singular EMG onset detection.

Maximum voluntary contraction (MVC) is a common scaling technique for EMG onset detection. MVC is the largest RMS amplitude a muscle generates in maximum contraction [31]. MVC has a curvilinear relationship with the muscle force production, where less force production amount to muscle weakness. EMG onset on a normalized time series with MVC can help diagnose gait disorders associated with atrophy [2]. Muscle spasticity/co-contraction during tremors among patients with neurological gait disorder exhibited abnormality in EMG onset compared to healthy individuals [12, 32]. EMG envelope indicated alterations in EMG onset for patients with Parkinson's during freezing episodes [20]. A premature activation of TA and GM muscles before a freezing episode was observed. In gait impairment, due to cervical spondylotic myelopathy, delayed onset and prolonged activation were present [12]. In cerebral palsy earlier onset suppression of EMG within cutaneous muscular reflex is associated with motor dysfunction, which results in inhibitory postsynaptic potentials [33].

4. EMG decomposition into MUAP

Raw EMG signal consists of superpositioned motor unit activation potentials (MUAP) and noise components. Muscle crosstalk is a major issue during recording of the biological signals. The crosstalk is dependent on factors such as anatomical site for the placement of electrodes, type of movement, and skin thickness. Since it is harder for sEMG to detect the origin of muscle electrical activity, the chances of muscle crosstalk are higher in sEMG than needle EMG [13]. Besides, low spatial resolution, high movement artifact, and narrow frequency range makes needle EMG more promising as a diagnostic tool in nerve conduction studies for assessing neurological disorders [13]. Changes in the shape of MUAPs, large dynamic range of action potential among motor units and superposition of motor units pose major challenges to decomposing the sEMG.

Fang et al. [34] decomposed EMG into MUAP by wavelet transform. The technique utilized spectrum matching in wavelet domain as opposed to waveform matching. De Luca et al. [35] proposed a method to decompose the sEMG into MUAP during cyclic dynamic contractions. The algorithm solved two main problems, the first associated with the displacement of the electrode on the surface of the skin leading to alteration in the shape of MUAPs, and second regarding lengthening and shortening of the muscle fibers while undergoing those contractions. The algorithm was an extension of the algorithm by Nawab et al. The process was followed as an extracting time-varying time template parameter, performing time-varying filter analysis, clustering on MUAP trains, shape refinement, test, and decomposition. If the test failed, the iterations were done again for shape refinement of MUAPs. Precision Decomposition I (PD I), which was earlier used to decompose needle EMG data was updated to decompose sEMG and referred as PD (III). An updated approach of PD III reported by Nawab et al. has PD-IPUS (Integrated Processing and Understanding) and PD-IGAT (Iterative Generate and Test) [36, 37]. Another method to decompose sEMG into MUAP trains included a hybrid approach of K-means clustering and convolution kernel compensation method. K-means clustering was performed to estimate the pulse trains, which were later updated iteratively by convolution kernel compensation method [38].

MUAP abnormality	Anatomical relation to changes
Increased amplitude	Increment in connective tissues, loss of muscle fibers
Decreased amplitude	Muscle fibers grouping
Decreased duration	Loss of muscle fibers
Increased duration	Increased muscle fibers
Increased spike duration	Variation in muscle diameter and increased endplate thickness
Increase in number of turns and phases	Slow conduction of terminal axons/increased diameter of muscle fiber and end plate
Increase in firing rate	Loss of motor units
Increase in the jiggle	Atypical neuromuscular transmission

Table 1.
MUAP abnormalities and indicated anatomical changes.

The question arises, what changes may a neurological disorder or injury bring to MUAPs? The features of a MUAP (rise time, duration, amplitude, phases/turns, recruitment and, stability) are vital to diagnosing the cause of abnormality in muscle coordination leading to gait or other movement disorders. A normal motor unit and a motor unit after injury (axonal injury) are distinguishable [32, 39–41]. MUAPs from needle EMG are not only adequate in diagnosing neuropathy (nerve injury) but can also determine the severity of the neuropathic condition [41]. Abnormal motor units constitute polyphasic potentials, unlike diphasic or triphasic potentials that exist in healthy individuals. Polyphasic potentials are a result of nascent potentials and terminal collateral sprouting [40]. Rodriguez-Carreno et al. [6] reported MUAPs shape abnormality pertinent to the anatomical phenomena shown in **Table 1**. A study conducted on mice with amyotrophic lateral sclerosis (ALS) using single unit extracellular recording within the spinal cord and EMG revealed gait variability [32]. In ALS mice, the low frequency of motor neuron and irregularities in the motor burst were co-occurring with fractionated EMG.

Among patients with myopathy, short, small, long duration, polyphasic and early recruitment of MUAPs were observed [39]. Different myopathy disorder studies in relation to MUAP trains were conducted using needle EMG by Paganoni et al. [39]. In early phases of disorders due to loss in muscle fibers the compound muscle action potential amplitude is lower. The result was short, small and early recruitment of MUAPs, but in Lambert-Eaton Myasthenic Syndrome, higher CMAP amplitude was observed. The shapes of MUAPs also alter with chronicity. Instead of positive sharp wave and fibrillation in the needle EMG, a mixture of long and short duration of EMG is prevalent [39]. Use of sEMG in comparison to needle EMG for postural disorder is preferable. sEMG is very good at detecting kinesiological disorders such as myotonia, myoclonus and tremors [13]. It can further be decomposed into MUAPs with the PD (III) algorithm, or hybrid of K-means and convolution kernel compensation method.

5. Extraction of muscle synergies

Linear decomposition of multi-source EMG signal is another method to diagnose the alteration in EMG patterns of patients with gait disorders [5, 42]. The muscle synergy hypothesis can be employed to understand better the physiological aspects of gait disorders using a number of linear decomposition algorithms such as principal component analysis (PCA), factor analysis (FA), independent component analysis (ICA), and non-negative matrix factorization algorithm (NNMF). Each algorithm is unique and extracts the synergy structure based on the assumption made on the synergy (e.g. orthogonality, non-negativity, statistical independence, etc.). After applying the factorization algorithm, the multi-electrode EMG signal is decomposed into the activation coefficients and synergies. The synergy vectors from the healthy group can be compared with a group suffering from the neurological or non-neurological disorder [43]. Statistical tests including cosine correlation, Pearson correlation or cluster analysis are generally used to compare the similarity and alterations in synergy structures [44, 45]. The application of a clustering algorithm for diagnosing gait disorder is discussed in a later section. Patients with thoracic spinal cord injury revealed lesser modules, higher co-contraction and, less directional tuning in relation to healthy individuals [46]. It is likely that the number of dimensional space was affected due to the choice of preprocessing [47]. A review cum research by Kieliba et al. [47] supported that increase in the cut off frequency of the filter decreases the variance, accounts for a particular component and increases dimensional space of synergies to be extracted. EMG acquired from children with cerebral palsy and from individual's post-stroke has shown that the choice of preprocessing (filtering, normalization) had an effect on the number of synergies and differentiation of physiological traits [48, 49]. **Figure 3** displays how the choice of low pass filter (10 and 20 Hz), a second-order Butterworth filter, effects the dimensional space. Filters are generally used to remove movement artifact. The principal component variance is higher for 10 than 20 Hz.

From a neurophysiological perspective, the recruitment of fewer spinal modules during movement is due to the loss of supraspinal inflow that results in simple muscle coordination (neuroadaptation). In upper extremities, the neuroadaptation was similarly perceived in the form of changes in the dimensional space of muscle synergy structures. Alteration of synergy structures was also present in patients with chronic stroke (upper extremity), and cerebral palsy [42, 43, 45, 50]. The linear envelopes extracted from the EMG data are subjected to MS extraction. The synergy hypothesis is well suited for capturing the physiological aspects of motor

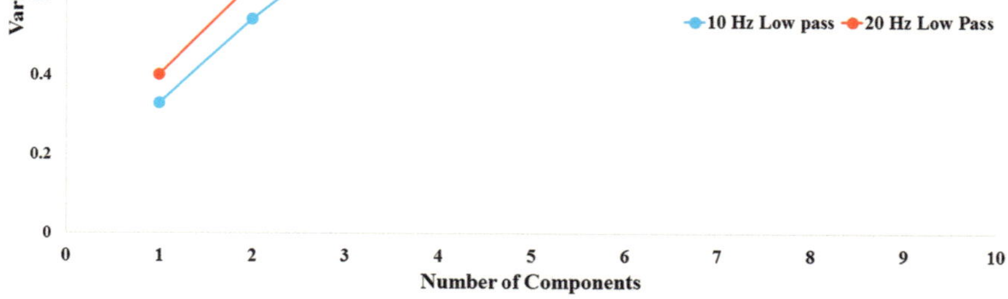

Figure 3.
A variance threshold ≥0.9 reveals five synergies for 10 Hz low pass filter and four synergies for 20 Hz low pass filter for 9-channel EMG data.

impairment [19]. In chronic stroke, merging and fractionation of synergies were observed. Merging of muscle synergies results in poor muscle coordination. In children with cerebral palsy, the dimensional space was smaller than it was in the control participants (unimpaired) [42]. However, the modules for cerebral palsy were higher for Duchenne muscular dystrophy (DMD) and typical developing (TD) children [43]. Rodriguez et al. revealed that fewer modules were recruited while walking on treadmill among Parkinson's patients. Thus, the size of dimensional space is crucial for the assessment of gait disorder such as cerebral palsy and Parkinson's [51, 52]. It is also important to properly choose preprocessing before analyzing the synergies as the dimensional space is sensitive to the preprocessing methods.

6. Frequency and time-frequency analysis

EMG power spectrum estimation methods can be categorized into parametric and nonparametric techniques. The spectral methods include fast Fourier transform (FFT), multitaper analysis and short-time Fourier transform (STFT) and wavelet transform. The difference between FFT and Wavelet Transformation is that FFT is localized to the frequency domain whereas the latter is localized to time-frequency analysis. Hu [53] recorded cortical and spinal somatosensory evoked potential (CSEP and SSEP), cortical motor evoked potential (CMEP) and spinal cord evoked potential (SCEP). The short time Fourier transformation was applied to the CSEP signal with a Hanning window [53]. The results revealed that the time-frequency analysis is a better marker for spinal injury than time domain analysis. The peak power after spinal injury had lesser energy with more dispersion in time-frequency scale.

The EMG time series signal can be analyzed in the frequency domain for the diagnosis of gait disorders. The frequency spectrum for EMG signals is in range of 0–500 Hz [54]. The FFT algorithm [55] computes the discrete Fourier transform (DFT) of EMG signal more efficiently. The FFT decomposes the EMG signals into periodic sine and cosine waves. We computed the FFT of EMG signal recorded from the Vastus Medialis (VM) during walking (**Figure 4**).

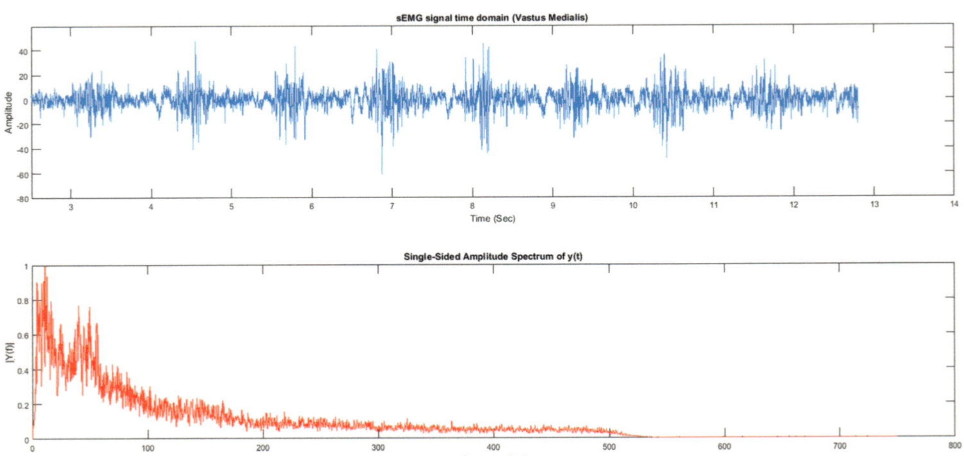

Figure 4.
(A) sEMG signal from VM during walking in time domain; (B) frequency domain representation of the signal using FFT.

The FFT allows computation of power spectra by squaring of FFT's magnitude [56]. In Parkinson disease, the spectral power of the signal has lower amplitude for the usual tremor than for the unusual tremor, which has peak amplitude of 4–6 Hz during an atypical tremor [15]. The signals associated with nonperiodic tremors are differentiable with FFT [57]. The EMG signal from neuropathic patients with SCI also exhibited distinct power spectrum density and amplitude in comparison to healthy individuals [58]. The application of FFT to the EMG envelope revealed muscle burst discharge in frequency domain ranging from 4 to 7 Hz [15]. Average power spectra computed from fractionated EMG of ALS mice by FFT was significantly higher than the control group. In the ALS group the spectra were skewed towards higher frequency content but single unit recordings revealed the absence of higher motor neuron (MN) frequencies or shortening of MN frequency in ALS mice [32], due to small type firing neurons improperly increasing firing frequency. This phenomenon results in co-contraction thus producing fractionated EMG. Co-contraction in muscles can also be observed in spinal cord injured patients [32]. In a study, EMG signals from lower limbs of dystonic and non-dystonic participants while walking were recorded. The non-dystonic participants were also patients suffering from other gait disorders. The power spectral density was computed using FFT with the Welch method of 50% overlap. The median power frequency (MdPF) and total power in low frequency were calculated for each muscle. The results revealed that MdPF for dystonic muscles had shifted to low frequencies and a concurrent increase in total power percentage in low-frequency range was observed [59]. Thus, frequency analysis of EMG signal not only provides us with distinction between normal and abnormal gait behavior but also specific gait abnormalities can be distinguished.

6.1 Short-time Fourier transform

Short-time Fourier transformation (STFT) is used to analyze a nonstationary signal in the frequency-domain. The signal is sliced and subjected to Fourier transform. Segmenting the signal is called time domain windowing, and the time localized signal is defined by $S_t(\tau) = S(\tau)h(\tau - t)$, where $h(t)$ is the window function centered at time t. The equation for STFT is given by (2).

$$S_t(\omega,t) = \frac{1}{\sqrt{2n}}\int S(\tau)h(\tau - t)e^{-i\omega t}.d\tau \tag{2}$$

Mitchell et al. [60] used cross time-frequency analysis to diagnose hypertension of the GM muscle. The study included 57 elderly people with 10 younger adults. Reduced Interference distribution (RID) was utilized to remove cross terms implementing time smoothing window and frequency smoothing window. A Hanning frequency smoothing window was chosen. In the study of gait, it is necessary to consider a time-localized cross-correlation between two signals, such as left and right muscle groups responsible for gait [60]. Hence, cross Wigner distribution (CWD) was selected to preserve the phase information. The results revealed statistical significance for several time-frequency parameters of sEMG between control group and persons with neuropathy, diabetes, osteoporosis, and arthritis patients [60]. STFT does not adopt an optimal time window or frequency resolution for non-stationary signals [7]. For the implementation of FFT and STFT the signals are considered to be stationary [8]. The problem or resolution can be overcome by continuous wavelet transform (CWT) [8]. Multitaper analysis is another and perhaps more efficient method for power spectral analysis to deal with non-stationary signals [61, 62].

6.2 The wavelet transform

Wavelet transform such as Multitaper is well suited for non-stationary signals. Wavelet transform elicits good localization of energy when the MUAP shape matches that of the wavelet [8]. Continuous wavelet transform (CWT) of bandpass filtered EMG showed alteration in the motor unit among stroke patients when a foot drop stimulator device was used (FDS) [63]. Energy localization below 100 Hz that resulted from foot drop was caused by slow motor unit recruitment. The neuromuscular activation improved with FDS. The time-frequency plot for Gastrocnemius showed that peak energy localization shifted from 50 to 100 Hz as a neuromuscular strategy [63]. Instantaneous mean frequency (IMNF) is the average frequency of power density spectrum of a signal and is computed from time-frequency distribution, $W(f, t)$ [63], where W is obtained from continuous wavelet transformation defined by (3) and (4).

$$IMNF(t) = \frac{\sum_{j=1}^{N} f_i W(f_i, t)}{\sum_{j=1}^{N} W(f_i, t)} \tag{3}$$

$$W(x,y) = \frac{1}{\sqrt{x}} \int_{-\infty}^{+\infty} y(t) \psi . \frac{(t-y)}{x} dt \tag{4}$$

In the above, x is the scaling factor that controls the width of the wavelet, y controls its location in time, ψ is the mother wavelet function and $y(t)$ is the signal. Instantaneous mean frequency can also be computed from the scalogram of CWT by its dimensional reduction. The scalogram has three dimensional space with time (x axis), frequency (y axis) and power (z axis) [63, 64]. In growing children, the higher IMNF level computed from scalogram revealed difference with respect to the children with cerebral palsy. The IMNF frequency component, unlike healthy children, decreased with age and maturation for children with cerebral palsy. IMNF also provided significant differences between the affected and unaffected site among stroke patients [63].

7. Feature extraction and classification

Time and frequency domain features of the EMG signal may be used to diagnose gait disorders. For example, an image processing technique can be used to detect pathological gait affected by abnormal firing of MUs [65]. Machine learning algorithms are important tools in detecting the pattern of normal and abnormal gait [66, 67]. They do so by making minimum assumptions about the data generating system, as it does not need a carefully controlled experimental design [9]. Application of machine learning algorithms to detect and classify gait disorders is suited to big data. Machine Learning is further divided into: (1) Supervised learning and (2) unsupervised learning. We will now discuss techniques to detect gait disorders using supervised and unsupervised learning algorithms.

7.1 Unsupervised learning

Unsupervised learning can be used to find structures in the EMG data. For example, cluster analysis has been used to identify alteration in the gait patterns, which are undetected by statistical tests. Patients with Parkinson's disease can be distinguished from a healthy individual by using cluster analysis of dimensionally reduced feature vector [68, 69]. K-means clustering is a very common clustering technique that initially estimates K centroids randomly or selectively. The algorithm iterates between two steps, data assignment steps and updating centroid. The aim is to minimize objective function, which is given by (5).

$$V(j) = \sum_{j=1}^{k}\sum_{i=1}^{n} ||x_i - c_j||^2 \quad (5)$$

where $V(j)$ is the objective function, n is the number of data points in jth cluster, k is the number of clusters and $||x_i - c_j||^2$ is the square of Euclidean distance.

The hypothesis of muscle synergies has been applied in several studies [44, 45, 70]. Unsupervised Learning helps in grouping identical synergies and can be helpful in diagnosing gait disorders. Kim et al. [70] identified synergies using iterative K-mean clustering and intraclass correlation. Hierarchical, model-based, fuzzy c means clustering has been employed to group gait patterns [69, 71–73]. Dolatabadi et al. [71] used mixture model clustering on spatiotemporal gait pattern to classify pathological gait. Pathological disorders such as cerebral palsy that show higher inter-stride variability can be analyzed with a hierarchical clustering method proposed by Rosati et al. [72]. Feature Fusion technique with Davies Bouldin Index (DBI) based on fuzzy C means algorithm was used in a trip/fall study [73]. The DBI can be used to evaluate the clustering algorithm. We have used K mean cluster analysis to cluster normal gait and gait with constraints, which are displayed in **Figure 5**.

7.2 Supervised learning

In supervised learning, the predictive models are based on the input and output data. Some of the widely used learning algorithms are decision trees, Bayesian networks, support vector machine, artificial neural networks, and linear discriminant analysis (LDA). After feature extraction and classification, the EMG time series can be modeled to control prosthetic or rehabilitative device. The fundamental approach to classification of EMG signal is shown in **Figure 6** [66].

The performance of different algorithms (SVM, LDA, MLP) in classifying gait disorders (Cerebral Palsy) was compared [74]. SVM classifier, compared to LDA and MLP, performed better when the analysis was done on kinematic data [74]. The normalization of the EMG data from different limb configurations increased

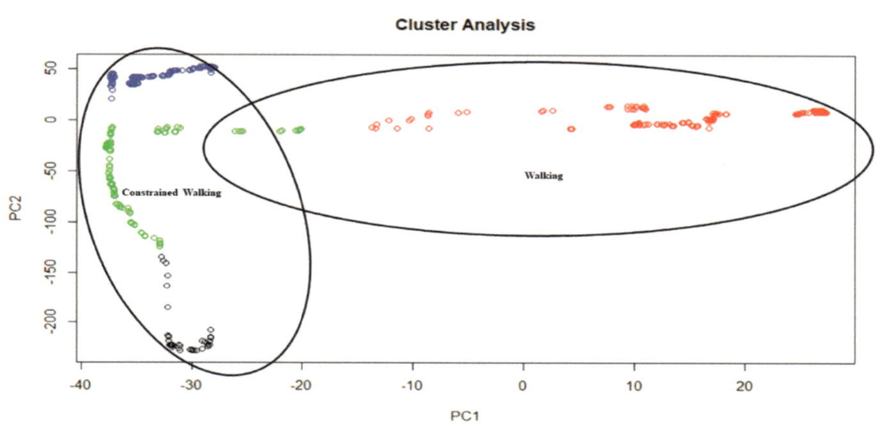

Figure 5.
A total of four clusters were chosen to group sEMG signal based on 93% variability in data within each cluster. The clusters were plotted for the first two principal components for walking with and without constraint.

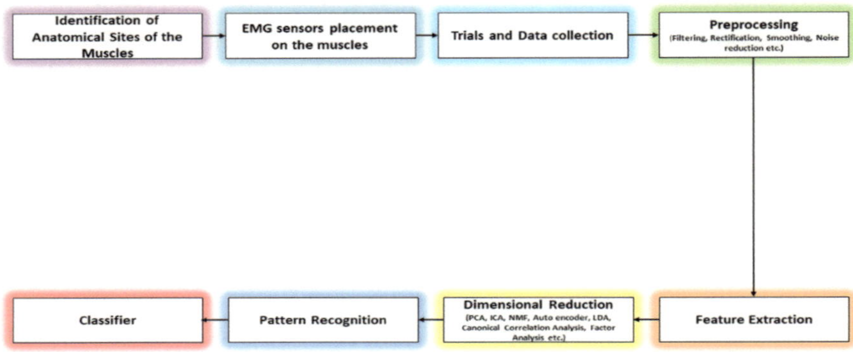

Figure 6.
Block diagram of an EMG Signal classification system.

classification accuracy [74, 75]. Feature level fusion is used to extract the feature space from daily life activities [73]. Patients with Parkinson's were classified with high accuracy using SVM with leave-one-out cross-validation [75]. Results from Nair et al. [76] suggest that least square kernel algorithm performed better than LDA, Neural Network, MLP and learning vector quantification (LVQ) for patients with arthritis. Decision Tree (DT) classifier used to classify toe walking gait disorder revealed three major toe-walking patterns [77]: (1) muscle weakness of TA and quadriceps and spasticity of Tibialis Surae; (2) severe spasticity of Tibialis Surae with limited range of ankle motion; and, (3) hamstring spasticity. The MLP, on the other hand, exhibited higher accuracy while classifying gait disorders associated with myopathy and neuropathy. Based on the literature studied, normalization, feature extraction and selection are important steps for accurately classifying gait disorders [75, 76].

Artificial neural networks (ANNs) are considered better at discovering nonlinear relationships in data. Ozsert et al. [78] classified biceps, frontalis and abductor muscles using ANN. The authors used wavelet transform for pre-processing the sEMG signal and an AR model to train the ANN. Senanayake et al. [79] used EMG RMS value and soft tissue deformation parameter (STDP) extracted from the video recordings to train a feed-forward-backward propagation neural network (FFBPN) to identify gait patterns. The proposed evaluation scheme improved classification accuracy between healthy and injured subject's gait patterns as Vastus Medialis and Lateralis revealed higher positive correlation between EMG and STDP for healthy individuals [79].

An adaptive neuro-fuzzy inference system (ANFIS) successfully diagnosed neurological disorders [8, 80]. In a number of studies, ANN and SVM worked well in diagnosing the gait pathology [7, 8, 71, 81]. Naik et al. [82] decomposed needle EMG from brachial biceps with ensemble empirical mode decomposition (EMD). The authors used Fast ICA and LDA classifier with majority voting to diagnose healthy participants from ALS, and myopathic individuals [82]. The algorithm of Naik et al. [83] for walking, sitting and standing tasks, achieved 86% classification accuracy for participants with and 96% without knee pathology. ICA via entropy bound minimization, time domain feature extraction, and feature selection with fisher score were performed prior to LDA classification. Ai et al. [30] used fused accelerometer and EMG data to discriminate among four participants including an amputee; more amputees in the study could provide better insight of the suggested technique [30].

There is no perfect machine learning algorithm to detect gait disorders. Signal processing techniques for feature extraction and selection, and standardization of the time series play a crucial role in enhancing classification accuracy. We also see consistent improvement in the existing models with increased classification accuracy [84]. ANN classifier has some deficiencies, such as high training process time and overfitting. Extreme Machine Learning algorithm (EML) improves on these anomalies at no cost to classification accuracy [8]. SVM accuracy was low for eight

Classifier	Authors	Year	Conditions	Classification	Performance
Neural networks	Senanayake et al.	2014	Soft tissue deformation	Gait pattern identification between healthy and injured	Accuracy = 98%
	Nair et al.	2010	Osteoarthritis	EMG of healthy and osteoarthritis	Accuracy = 89.4 ± 11.8%
	Nair et al.	2010	Rheumatoid arthritis	EMG of healthy and rheumatoid arthritis	Accuracy = 57 ± 1 8%
	Kamruzzaman and Begg.	2006	Cerebral palsy	Gait pattern identification using stride length and cadence	Accuracy = 94.87%
LDA	Naik et al.	2018	Knee pathology	Movement classification for healthy and patients with knee pathology	Accuracy = 86% (Unhealthy) and 96% (Healthy)
	Nair et al.	2010	Rheumatoid arthritis	EMG of healthy and rheumatoid arthritis	Accuracy = 72 ± 20%
	Ai et al.	2017	Normal and amputated	Movement-based classification for normal and amputee subject	Accuracy = 95.6 ± 2.2%
	Kamruzzaman and Begg.	2006	Cerebral palsy	Gait pattern identification using stride length and cadence	Accuracy = 93.59%
SVM	Kamruzzaman and Begg.	2006	Cerebral palsy	Gait pattern identification using stride length and cadence	Accuracy = 96.8%
	Kugler et al.	2013	Parkinson	Differentiate between healthy and Parkinson patients by auto-step segmentation	Specificity = 90% and Sensitivity = 90%
	Ai et al.	2017	Normal and amputated	Movement-based classification for normal and amputee subject	Accuracy = 98.1 ± 1.6%
	Xi et al.	2018	Fall	Gait recognition for daily life activities including Fall	Accuracy = 100%
Decision tree	Armand et al.	2006	Toe Walking disorders	Identification of ankle kinematic patterns for toe walkers	Accuracy = 81%

Classifier	Authors	Year	Conditions	Classification	Performance
Least square Kernel Algorithm	Nair et al.	2010	Rheumatoid arthritis	EMG of healthy and rheumatoid arthritis	Accuracy = 91%
	Nair et al.	2010	Osteoarthritis	EMG of healthy and osteoarthritis	Accuracy = 97%

Table 2.
EMG classification methods.

daily life activities including falling. The accuracy for detecting trip fall improved with weighted genetic algorithm [73]. A wide variety of time domain, frequency domain, and time-frequency domain features, and optimization techniques provide multiple options to enhance the classification accuracy of gait diagnosis. The performance of each algorithmic class discussed in this review with respect to the abnormal physiological condition is shown in **Table 2**.

8. Future trends

The computational methods reviewed in this study have evolved over several decades and continue to do so. For example, ANOVA test's inability to detect visually observable waveform due to abnormal gait behavior had been improved with wfANOVA test [20]. Apart from factorization algorithms and PCA, artificial neural

EMG method	Pros	Cons
Visual inspection of raw EMG	1. Lower computational burden 2. Takes advantage of experience	1. Relies on experience only, hence chances of error 2. Limited theoretical basis
EMG envelope/ onset detection	1. EMG onset can reveal altered muscle activity (e.g., freezing episodes in Parkinson's)	1. Impacted by a number of parameters, hence may not be reliable
Frequency and time-frequency analysis	1. Provides quantitative information in frequency and time-frequency domain 2. Specific Gait abnormalities can be distinguished (suitable for SCI patients) 3. Provides additional features like MdPF, IMNF for further classification 4. Provides algorithmic options that sidestep stationarity issues	1. Added processing time and computational burden 2. Assumption of stationarity is made for some FFT tools
MUAP decomposition	1. An abnormality in MUAP's shape reveals altered motor behavior 2. Requires less processing for Needle EMG	1. Harder to decompose sEMG signal 2. Computational cost is high for sEMG
Muscle synergy decomposition	1. Recovers dominant spatio-temporal profiles in EMG signal 2. Useful in certain disorder diagnosis (Cerebral Palsy, stroke, SCI, etc.) 3. Computational cost is dependent on the type of factorization algorithm	1. Preprocessing of EMG signal impacts the dimensional space for synergy extraction 2. Choice of algorithm alters the results, i.e., assumption on the type of synergies need to be made

Table 3.
Pros and cons of EMG processing techniques discussed.

network were implemented for synergy extraction [5]. New time and frequency domain features and hybrid methods for feature selection have been developed and introduced over the years [67]. In these examples, the conventional techniques were enhanced or detection of gait disorders. There is a consistent effort to augment current computational techniques and improve the EMG based detection methods for motor behavior abnormalities. Optimization algorithms, feature level fusion, and advances in computational methodology point to a future for detecting intricate EMG patterns EMG associated with abnormal gait behavior in machine learning. Recently, application of deep learning algorithms to detect abnormal EMG patterns appears more promising [85], and performs well with EMG acquired directly from the muscles. The main issue in clinical application of deep learning is its real-time implementation. The development of powerful graphics processing unit (GPU) and faster training algorithms will likely resolve such issues in near future.

In conclusion, in this article we reviewed the existing literature on EMG processing techniques from simple thresholding to complex computation algorithms and their application in detecting gait disorders. The pros and cons of the techniques discussed are summarized in **Table 3**. Besides discussing these techniques in detail, our study cites pertinent literature where these techniques were successfully used to detect gait abnormalities. This study clearly points towards the recent trend in assessing gait disorders from EMG data using an intelligent system. Examples of such systems using supervised and unsupervised learning were also reviewed.

Author details

Rajat Emanuel Singh[1], Kamran Iqbal[1]*, Gannon White[2] and Jennifer K. Holtz[2]

1 College of Engineering and Information Technology, University of Arkansas at Little Rock, Arkansas, USA

2 School of Counseling, Human Performance, and Rehabilitation, University of Arkansas at Little Rock, Arkansas, USA

*Address all correspondence to: kxiqbal@ualr.edu

References

[1] Luca CJ. Physiology and mathematics of myoelectric signals. IEEE Transactions on Biomedical Engineering, BME. 1979;**26**(6):313-325. DOI: 10.1109/tbme.1979.326534

[2] Konard P. The ABC of EMG: A Practical Introduction to Kinesiological Electromyography. USA: Noeraxon Inc.; 2005. Version 1.0

[3] Luca CJ. The Wartenweiler memorial lecture the use of surface electromyography in biomechanics. Journal of Biomechanics. 1994;**27**(6):724. DOI: 10.1016/0021-9290(94)91124-x

[4] Stifani N. Motor neurons and the generation of spinal motor neuron diversity. Frontiers in Cellular Neuroscience. 2014;**8**:293. DOI: 10.3389/fncel.2014.00293

[5] Singh RE, Iqbal K, White G, Hutchinson TE. A systematic review on muscle synergies: From building blocks of motor behavior to a neurorehabilitation tool. Applied Bionics and Biomechanics. 2018;**2018**:3615368. DOI: 10.1155/2018/3615368

[6] Rodriguez-Carreno I, Gila-Useros L, Malanda-Trigueros A. Motor unit action potential duration: measurement and significance. In: Ajeena I editor. Advances in Clinical Neurophysiology, ISBN: 978-953-51-0806-1, Ch 7. 2012. DOI: 10.5772/50265

[7] Raez MBI, Hussain MS, Mohd-Yasin F. Techniques of EMG signal analysis: detection, processing, classification and applications. Biological Procedures Online. 2006;**8**:11-35. DOI: 10.1251/bpo115

[8] Chowdhury RH, Reaz MBI, Ali MABM, Bakar AAA, Chellappan K, Chang TG. Surface electromyography signal processing and classification techniques. Sensors (Basel, Switzerland). 2013;**13**(9):12431-12466. DOI: 10.3390/s130912431

[9] Bzdok D, Altman N, Krzywinski M. Points of significance: Statistics versus machine learning. Nature Methods. 2018;**15**(4):233-234. DOI: 10.1038/nmeth.4642

[10] Iniesta R, Stahl D, McGuffin P. Machine learning, statistical learning and the future of biological research in psychiatry. Psychological Medicine. 2016;**46**(12):2455-2465. DOI: 10.1017/S0033291716001367

[11] Dietz V. Degradation of neuronal function following a spinal cord injury: Mechanisms and countermeasures. Brain. 2004;**127**(10):2221-2231. DOI: 10.1093/brain/awh255

[12] Malone A, Meldrum D, Gleeson J, Bolger C. Electromyographic characteristics of gait impairment in cervical spondylotic myelopathy. European Spine Journal. 2013;**22**(11):2538-2544. DOI: 10.1007/s00586-013-2928-9

[13] Pullman SL, Goodin DS, Marquinez AI, Tabbal S, Rubin M. Clinical utility of surface EMG: report of the therapeutics and technology assessment subcommittee of the American Academy of Neurology. Neurology. 2000;**55**:171-177

[14] Burridge J, Wood D, Taylor P, Mclellan D. Indices to describe different muscle activation patterns, identified during treadmill walking, in people with spastic drop-foot. Medical Engineering & Physics. 2001;**23**(6):427-434. DOI: 10.1016/s1350-4533(01)00061-3

[15] Perumal SV, Sankar R. Gait monitoring system for patients with Parkinsons disease using wearable sensors. In: 2016 IEEE Healthcare

Innovation Point-Of-Care Technologies Conference (HI-POCT). 2016. DOI: 10.1109/hic.2016.7797687

[16] Domingo A, Sawicki GS, Ferris DP. Kinematics and muscle activity of individuals with incomplete spinal cord injury during treadmill stepping with and without manual assistance. Journal of Neuroengineering and Rehabilitation. 2007;**4**:32. DOI: 10.1186/1743-0003-4-32

[17] Banks CL, Huang HJ, Little VL, Patten C. Electromyography exposes heterogeneity in muscle co-contraction following stroke. Frontiers in Neurology. 2017;**8**:699. DOI: 10.3389/fneur.2017.00699

[18] Nieuwboer A, Dom R, Weerdt WD, Desloovere K, Janssens L, Stijn V. Electromyographic profiles of gait prior to onset of freezing episodes in patients with Parkinsons disease. Brain. 2004;**127**(7):1650-1660. DOI: 10.1093/brain/awh189

[19] Lukhanina E, Karaban I, Berezetskay N. Diagnosis of Parkinsons disease by electrophysiological methods. In: Dushanova J editor. Diagnostics and Rehabilitation of Parkinsons Disease, Ch 2. 2011. DOI: 10.5772/17761

[20] McKay JL, Welch TDJ, Vidakovic B, Ting LH. Statistically significant contrasts between EMG waveforms revealed using wavelet-based functional ANOVA. Journal of Neurophysiology. 2013;**109**(2):591-602. DOI: 10.1152/jn.00447.2012

[21] PhysioNet. Available online: http://www.physionet.org [Accessed: July 1, 2018]

[22] Bar-On L, Aertbeliën E, Molenaers G, Desloovere K. Muscle activation patterns when passively stretching spastic lower limb muscles of children with cerebral palsy. PLoS One. 2014;**9**(3):e91759. DOI: 10.1371/journal.pone.0091759

[23] Morey-Klapsing G, Arampatzis A, Brüggemann GP. Choosing EMG parameters: Comparison of different onset determination algorithms and EMG integrals in a joint stability study. Clinical Biomechanics. 2004;**19**(2):196-201. DOI: 10.1016/j.clinbiomech.2003.10.010

[24] Solnik S, DeVita P, Rider P, Long B, Hortobágyi T. Teager–Kaiser operator improves the accuracy of EMG onset detection independent of signal-to-noise ratio. Acta of Bioengineering and Biomechanics/Wroclaw University of Technology. 2008;**10**(2):65-68

[25] Tenan MS, Tweedell AJ, Haynes CA. Analysis of statistical and standard algorithms for detecting muscle onset with surface electromyography. PLoS One. 2017;**12**(5):e0177312. DOI: 10.1371/journal.pone.0177312

[26] Staude G, Flachenecker C, Daumer M, Wolf W. Onset detection in surface electromyographic signals: A systematic comparison of methods. EURASIP Journal on Advances in Signal Processing. 2001;**2001**(2):867853. DOI: 10.1155/s1110865701000191

[27] Hodges P. A comparison of computer-based methods for the determination of onset of muscle contraction using electromyography. Electroencephalography and Clinical Neurophysiology. 1996;**101**(6):511-519. DOI: 10.1016/s0013-4694(96)95190-5

[28] Bonato P, Dalessio T, Knaflitz M. A statistical method for the measurement of muscle activation intervals from surface myoelectric signal during gait. IEEE Transactions on Biomedical Engineering. 1998;**45**(3):287-299. DOI: 10.1109/10.661154

[29] Lidierth M. A computer based method for automated measurement of the periods of muscular activity from an EMG and its application to locomotor EMGs. Electroencephalography

and Clinical Neurophysiology. 1986;**64**(4):378-380. DOI: 10.1016/0013-4694(86)90163-x

[30] Ai Q, Zhang Y, Qi W, Liu Q, Chen AK. Research on lower limb motion recognition based on fusion of sEMG and accelerometer signals. Symmetry. 2017;**9**(8):147. DOI: 10.3390/sym9080147

[31] Amplitude Analysis: Normalization of EMG to Maximum Voluntary Contraction (MVC). May 09, 2017. Retrieved from: https://www.delsys.com/emgworks-analysis-techniques-using-emgscript/

[32] Hadzipasic M, Ni W, Nagy M, Steenrod N, McGinley MJ, Kaushal A, et al. Reduced high-frequency motor neuron firing, EMG fractionation, and gait variability in awake walking ALS mice. Proceedings of the National Academy of Sciences of the United States of America. 2016;**113**(47):E7600-E7609. DOI: 10.1073/pnas.1616832113

[33] Condliffe EG, Jeffery DT, Emery DJ, Gorassini MA. Spinal inhibition and motor function in adults with spastic cerebral palsy. The Journal of Physiology. 2016;**594**(10):2691-2705. DOI: 10.1113/JP271886

[34] Fang J, Agarwal G, Shahani B. Decomposition of EMG signal by wavelet spectrum matching. In: Proceedings of the 19th Annual International Conference of the IEEE Engineering in Medicine and Biology Society. Magnificent Milestones and Emerging Opportunities in Medical Engineering (Cat. No.97CH36136). 1997. DOI: 10.1109/iembs.1997.756598

[35] De Luca CJ, Chang S-S, Roy SH, Kline JC, Nawab SH. Decomposition of surface EMG signals from cyclic dynamic contractions. Journal of Neurophysiology. 2015;**113**(6):1941-1951. DOI: 10.1152/jn.00555.2014

[36] Nawab SH, Chang S-S, De Luca CJ. High-yield decomposition of surface EMG signals. Clinical Neurophysiology: Official Journal of the International Federation of Clinical Neurophysiology. 2010;**121**(10):1602-1615. DOI: 10.1016/j.clinph.2009.11.092

[37] Luca CJ, Adam A, Wotiz R, Gilmore LD, Nawab SH. Decomposition of surface EMG signals. Journal of Neurophysiology. 2006;**96**(3):1646-1657. DOI: 10.1152/jn.00009.2006

[38] Ning Y, Zhu X, Zhu S, Zhang Y. Surface EMG decomposition based on K-means clustering and convolution kernel compensation. IEEE Journal of Biomedical and Health Informatics. 2015;**19**(2):471-477. DOI: 10.1109/JBHI.2014.2328497

[39] Paganoni S, Amato A. Electrodiagnostic evaluation of myopathies. Physical Medicine and Rehabilitation Clinics of North America. 2013;**24**(1):193-207. DOI: 10.1016/j.pmr.2012.08.017

[40] Feinberg J. EMG: Myths and facts. HSS Journal. 2006;**2**(1):19-21. DOI: 10.1007/s11420-005-0124-0

[41] Chung T, Prasad K, Lloyd TE. Peripheral neuropathy—Clinical and electrophysiological considerations. Neuroimaging Clinics of North America. 2014;**24**(1):49-65. DOI: 10.1016/j.nic.2013.03.023

[42] Steele KM, Rozumalski A, Schwartz MH. Muscle synergies and complexity of neuromuscular control during gait in cerebral palsy. Developmental Medicine and Child Neurology. 2015;**57**(12):1176-1182. DOI: 10.1111/dmcn.12826

[43] Goudriaan M, Shuman BR, Steele KM, Van den Hauwe M, Goemans N, Molenaers G, et al. Non-neural muscle weakness has limited influence on complexity of motor control during gait. Frontiers in Human

Neuroscience. 2018;**12**:5. DOI: 10.3389/fnhum.2018.00005

[44] Cheung VCK, Piron L, Agostini M, Silvoni S, Turolla A, Bizzi E. Stability of muscle synergies for voluntary actions after cortical stroke in humans. Proceedings of the National Academy of Sciences of the United States of America. 2009;**106**(46):19563-19568. DOI: 10.1073/pnas.0910114106

[45] Roh J, Rymer WZ, Beer RF. Evidence for altered upper extremity muscle synergies in chronic stroke survivors with mild and moderate impairment. Frontiers in Human Neuroscience. 2015;**9**:6. DOI: 10.3389/fnhum.2015.00006

[46] Milosevic M, Yokoyama H, Grangeon M, Masani K, Popovic MR, Nakazawa K, et al. Muscle synergies reveal impaired trunk muscle coordination strategies in individuals with thoracic spinal cord injury. Journal of Electromyography and Kinesiology. 2017;**36**:40-48. DOI: 10.1016/j.jelekin.2017.06.007

[47] Kieliba P, Tropea P, Pirondini E, Coscia M, Micera S, Artoni F. How are muscle synergies affected by electromyography pre-processing? IEEE Transactions on Neural Systems and Rehabilitation Engineering. 2018;**26**(4):882-893. DOI: 10.1109/tnsre.2018.2810859

[48] Banks CL, Pai MM, McGuirk TE, Fregly BJ, Patten C. Methodological choices in muscle synergy analysis impact differentiation of physiological characteristics following stroke. Frontiers in Computational Neuroscience. 2017;**11**:78. DOI: 10.3389/fncom.2017.00078

[49] Shuman BR, Schwartz MH, Steele KM. Electromyography data processing impacts muscle synergies during gait for unimpaired children and children with cerebral palsy. Frontiers in Computational Neuroscience. 2017;**11**:50. DOI: 10.3389/fncom.2017.00050

[50] Roh J, Rymer WZ, Perreault EJ, Yoo SB, Beer RF. Alterations in upper limb muscle synergy structure in chronic stroke survivors. Journal of Neurophysiology. 2013;**109**(3):768-781. DOI: 10.1152/jn.00670.2012

[51] Tang L, Li F, Cao S, Zhang X, Wu D, Chen X. Muscle synergy analysis in children with cerebral palsy. Journal of Neural Engineering. 2015;**12**:046017. DOI: 10.1088/1741-2560/12/4/046017

[52] Rodriguez KL, Roemmich RT, Cam B, Fregly BJ, Hass CJ. Persons with Parkinson's disease exhibit decreased neuromuscular complexity during gait. Clinical Neurophysiology: Official Journal of the International Federation of Clinical Neurophysiology. 2013;**124**(7):1390-1397. DOI: 10.1016/j.clinph.2013.02.006

[53] Hu Y. Prevention of spinal cord injury with time-frequency analysis of evoked potentials: An experimental study. Journal of Neurology, Neurosurgery & Psychiatry. 2001;**71**(6):732-740. DOI: 10.1136/jnnp.71.6.732

[54] DeLuca CJ. Fundamental Concepts in SEMG signal Acquisition. DelSys Inc Tutorial; 2003. https://delsys.com/Attachments_pdf/download/tutorials/01_fundamental-concepts-in-emg-signal-acquisition.pdf (accessed on 25 Dec 2018)

[55] Good IJ. Introduction to Cooley and Tukey (1965). An algorithm for the machine calculation of complex Fourier series. In: Kotz S and Johnson N editor. Breakthroughs in Statistics Vol III. New York: Springer; 1997. pp. 201-216. DOI: 10.1007/978-1-4612-0667-5_9

[56] Press WH et al. Sec. 13.4: Power spectrum estimation using the FFT. In:

Numerical Recipes in C. 2nd ed. New York: Cambridge University Press; 1992

[57] Grimaldi G, Manto M. Neurological tremor: Sensors, signal processing and emerging applications. Sensors. 2010;**10**(2):1399-1422. DOI: 10.3390/s100201399

[58] Sadikoglu F, Kavalcioglu C, Dagman B. Electromyogram (EMG) signal detection, classification of EMG signals and diagnosis of neuropathy muscle disease. Procedia Computer Science. 2017;**120**:422-429. DOI: 10.1016/j.procs.2017.11.259

[59] Go SA, Coleman-Wood K, Kaufman KR. Frequency analysis of lower extremity electromyography signals for the quantitative diagnosis of dystonia. Journal of Electromyography and Kinesiology: Official Journal of the International Society of Electrophysiological Kinesiology. 2014;**24**(1):31-36. DOI: 10.1016/j.jelekin.2013.11.002

[60] Mitchell P, Krotish D, Shin Y, Hirth V. Cross time-frequency analysis of gastrocnemius electromyographic signals in hypertensive and nonhypertensive subjects. EURASIP Journal on Advances in Signal Processing. 2010;**2010**(1):206560. DOI: 10.1155/2010/206560

[61] Babadi B, Brown EN. A review of multitaper spectral analysis. IEEE Transactions on Biomedical Engineering. 2014;**61**(5):1555-1564. DOI: 10.1109/tbme.2014.2311996

[62] Van Vugt MK, Sederberg PB, Kahana MJ. Comparison of spectral analysis methods for characterizing brain oscillations. Journal of Neuroscience Methods. 2007;**162**(1-2):49-63. DOI: 10.1016/j.jneumeth.2006.12.004

[63] Pilkar R, Ramanujam A, Nolan KJ. Alterations in spectral attributes of surface electromyograms after utilization of a foot drop stimulator during post-stroke gait. Frontiers in Neurology. 2017;**8**:449. DOI: 10.3389/fneur.2017.00449

[64] Lauer RT, Pierce SR, Tucker CA, Barbe MF, Prosser LA. Age and electromyographic frequency alterations during walking in children with cerebral palsy. Gait & Posture. 2010;**31**(1):136. DOI: 10.1016/j.gaitpost.2009.09.015

[65] Ren X, Huang H, Deng L. MUAP classification based on wavelet packet and fuzzy clustering technique. In: 2009 3rd International Conference on Bioinformatics and Biomedical Engineering. 2009. DOI: 10.1109/icbbe.2009.5163091

[66] Nazmi N, Abdul Rahman MA, Yamamoto S-I, Ahmad SA, Zamzuri H, Mazlan SA. A review of classification techniques of EMG signals during isotonic and isometric contractions. Sensors (Basel, Switzerland). 2016;**16**(8):1304. DOI: 10.3390/s16081304

[67] Mwadulo MW. A review on feature selection methods for classification tasks. International Journal of Computer Applications Technology and Research. 2016;**5**(6):395-402. DOI: 10.7753/ijcatr0506.1013

[68] Rissanen SM, Kankaanpää M, Meigal A, Tarvainen MP, Nuutinen J, Tarkka IM, et al. Surface EMG and acceleration signals in Parkinson's disease: Feature extraction and cluster analysis. Medical & Biological Engineering & Computing. 2008;**46**(9):849-858. DOI: 10.1007/s11517-008-0369-0

[69] Mulroy S, Gronley J, Weiss W, Newsam C, Perry J. Use of cluster analysis for gait pattern classification of patients in the early and late recovery phases following stroke. Gait & Posture. 2003;**18**(1):114-125. DOI: 10.1016/s0966-6362(02)00165-0

[70] Kim Y, Bulea TC, Damiano DL. Novel methods to enhance precision and reliability in muscle synergy identification during walking. Frontiers in Human Neuroscience. 2016;**10**:455. DOI: 10.3389/fnhum.2016.00455

[71] Dolatabadi E, Mansfield A, Patterson KK, Taati B, Mihailidis A. Mixture-model clustering of pathological gait patterns. IEEE Journal of Biomedical and Health Informatics. 2016;**5**:1297-1305. DOI: 10.1109/JBHI.2016.2633000

[72] Rosati S, Agostini V, Knaflitz M, Balestra G. Muscle activation patterns during gait: A hierarchical clustering analysis. Biomedical Signal Processing and Control. 2017;**31**:463-469. DOI: 10.1016/j.bspc.2016.09.017

[73] Xi X, Tang M, Luo Z. Feature-level fusion of surface electromyography for activity monitoring. Sensors. 2018;**18**(2):614. DOI: 10.3390/s18020614

[74] Kamruzzaman J, Begg R. Support vector machines and other pattern recognition approaches to the diagnosis of cerebral palsy gait. IEEE Transactions on Biomedical Engineering. 2006;**53**(12):2479-2490. DOI: 10.1109/tbme.2006.883697

[75] Kugler P, Jaremenko C, Schlachetzki J, Winkler J, Klucken J, Eskofier B. Automatic recognition of Parkinsons disease using surface electromyography during standardized gait tests. In: 2013 35th Annual International Conference of the IEEE Engineering in Medicine and Biology Society (EMBC). 2013. DOI: 10.1109/embc.2013.6610865

[76] Nair SS, French RM, Laroche D, Thomas E. The application of machine learning algorithms to the analysis of electromyographic patterns from arthritic patients. IEEE Transactions on Neural Systems and Rehabilitation Engineering. 2010;**18**(2):174-184. DOI: 10.1109/tnsre.2009.2032638

[77] Armand S, Watelain E, Roux E, Mercier M, Lepoutre F. Linking clinical measurements and kinematic gait patterns of toe-walking using fuzzy decision trees. Gait & Posture. 2007;**25**(3):475-484. DOI: 10.1016/j.gaitpost.2006.05.014

[78] Ozsert M, Yavuz O, Durak-Ata L. Analysis and classification of compressed EMG signals by wavelet transform via alternative neural networks algorithms. Computer Methods in Biomechanics and Biomedical Engineering. 2011;**14**(6):521-525. DOI: 10.1080/10255842.2010.485130

[79] Senanayake SM, Triloka J, Malik OA, Iskandar M. Artificial neural network based gait patterns identification using neuromuscular signals and soft tissue deformation analysis of lower limbs muscles. In: 2014 International Joint Conference on Neural Networks (IJCNN). 2014. DOI: 10.1109/ijcnn.2014.6889899

[80] Khezri M, Jahed M. A neuro-fuzzy inference system for sEMG-based identification of hand motion commands. IEEE Transactions on Industrial Electronics. 2011;**58**(5):1952-1960. DOI: 10.1109/tie.2010.2053334

[81] Xie H-B, Guo T, Bai S, Dokos S. Hybrid soft computing systems for electromyographic signals analysis: A review. Biomedical Engineering Online. 2014;**13**:8. DOI: 10.1186/1475-925X-13-8

[82] Naik GR, Selvan SE, Nguyen HT. Single-channel EMG classification with ensemble-empirical-mode-decomposition-based ICA for diagnosing neuromuscular disorders. IEEE Transactions on Neural Systems and Rehabilitation Engineering. 2016;**24**(7):734-743. DOI: 10.1109/tnsre.2015.2454503

[83] Naik GR, Selvan SE, Arjunan SP, Acharyya A, Kumar DK, Ramanujam A,

et al. An ICA-EBM-based sEMG classifier for recognizing lower limb movements in individuals with and without knee pathology. IEEE Transactions on Neural Systems and Rehabilitation Engineering. 2018;**26**(3):675-686. DOI: 10.1109/tnsre.2018.2796070

[84] Singh RE et al. Gait phase discrimination during kinematically constrained walking on slackline. Accepted in IEEE International Conference on Control and Automation. July 16-19, 2019, Edinburgh, Scotland

[85] Phinyomark A, Scheme E. EMG pattern recognition in the era of big data and deep learning. Big Data and Cognitive Computing. 2018;**2**(3):21. DOI: 10.3390/bdcc2030021

Chapter 3

Radiation Oncology in the Era of Big Data and Machine Learning for Precision Medicine

Alexander F.I. Osman

Abstract

Machine learning (ML) applications in medicine represent an emerging field of research with the potential to revolutionize the field of radiation oncology, in particular. With the era of big data, the utilization of machine learning algorithms in radiation oncology research is growing fast with applications including patient diagnosis and staging of cancer, treatment simulation, treatment planning, treatment delivery, quality assurance, and treatment response and outcome predictions. In this chapter, we provide the interested reader with an overview of the ongoing advances and cutting-edge applications of state-of-the-art ML techniques in radiation oncology process from the radiotherapy workflow perspective, starting from patient's diagnosis to follow-up. We present with discussion the areas where ML has presently been used and also areas where ML could be applied to improve the efficiency (i.e., optimizing and automating the clinical processes) and quality (i.e., potentials for decision-making support toward a practical application of precision medicine in radiation therapy) of patient care.

Keywords: big data, machine learning, radiation oncology, decision-making, precision medicine

1. Introduction

Radiation oncology is the discipline dealing with the treatment of malignant neoplasias or cancerous lesions (and occasionally benign lesions) with ionizing radiation for cure or palliation intent. The clinical modality or technique has been used to treat the patient in radiation oncology is referred to as radiation therapy (or "radiotherapy"). Radiotherapy has often given in combination with other treatment modalities for instance chemotherapy, surgery, hormonal therapy, etc. The aim of radiotherapy is to deliver a precisely measured dose of irradiation to a defined tumor volume with as minimal damage as possible to surrounding healthy tissue, resulting in eradication the tumor, high quality of life, and prolongation of survival [1]. **Figure 1** presents a typical radiotherapy workflow, from patient consult and assessment to follow-up. The field of radiotherapy has witnessed with significant technological advances over the last decades. This advancing has introduced the complexity of radiotherapy processes and generating a massive amount of data (also so-called "big data") during radiotherapy workflow.

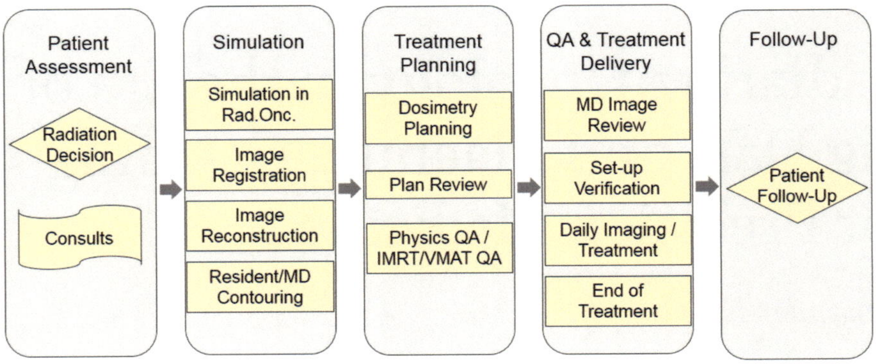

Figure 1.
Radiotherapy workflow, from patient consult and assessment to follow-up.

1.1 Big data

Big data is data which is of a large volume, often combining multiple data sets and requiring innovative forms of information technology to process this data [3]. Big data has characterized by four V's: volume, variety, velocity and veracity [3]. In radiation oncology, data can be categorized as "Big Data" because (a) the use of data-intensive imaging modalities (volume), (b) the imaging archives are growing rapidly (velocity), (c) there is an increasing amount of imaging and diagnostic modalities available (variety), and (d) interpretation and quality differs between care providers (veracity) [4]. The radiation oncologists are overwhelmed with scientific literature, rapidly evolving treatment techniques, and the exponentially increasing amount of clinical data [5]. **Figure 2** shows more and more information is associated with the patient as the proceeds along the radiotherapy process, like a snowball rolling down a hill [2]. The radiation oncologists need help translating all these data into knowledge that supports decision-making in routine clinical practice [6–10].

In this direction, such collaborative efforts have been established in the last few years to advance the possibilities of using big data to facilitate personalized clinical patient care in the field of radiation oncology. For example, in 2015, the American Society for Therapeutic Radiation Oncology (ASTRO), National Cancer Institute (NCI), and American Association of Physicists in Medicine (AAPM) co-organized a workshop with aims focused on opportunities for radiation oncology in the era of big data [9]. Later in 2017, the American College of Radiology (ACR) has established the Data Science Institute (DSI) with a core purpose to empower the advancement, validation, and implementation of artificial intelligence (AI) in medical imaging and the radiological science for the benefit of patients, society, and the profession [10].

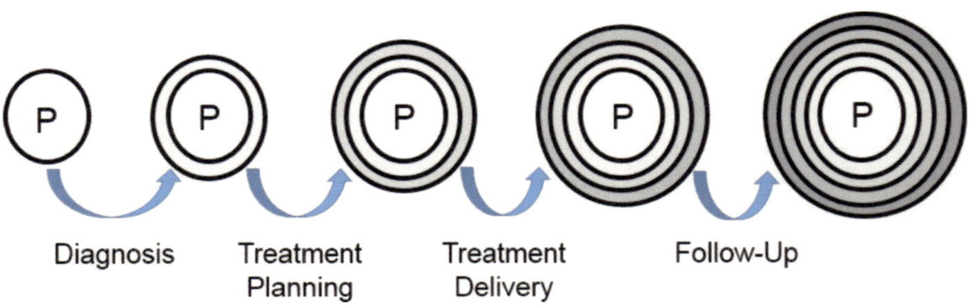

Figure 2.
With each step along the radiotherapy workflow, more information is created and collected which has associated with the patient (reproduced from [2]).

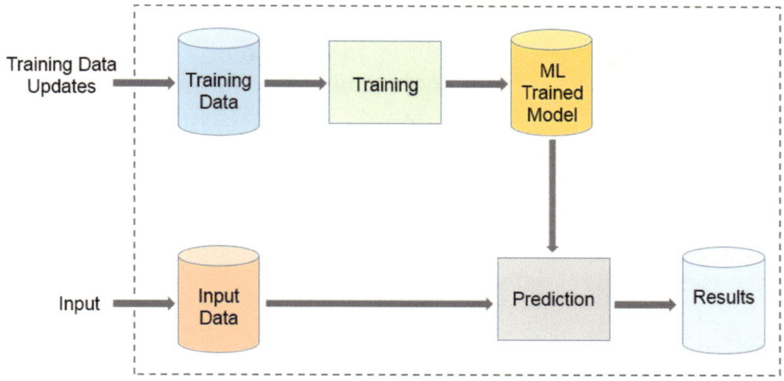

Figure 3.
A generic machine learning workflow.

1.2 Machine learning

Machine learning (ML), a branch of artificial intelligence, is the technology of developing computer algorithms that are able to emulate human intelligence. An ML algorithm is a computational process that uses input data to achieve the desired task without being literally programmed (i.e., "hard-coded") to produce a particular outcome [2]. These algorithms are in a sense "soft-coded" in that they automatically alter or adapt their architecture through repetition (i.e., experience) so that they become better and better at achieving the desired task [2]. The process of adaptation is called training, in which samples of input data have provided along with desired outcomes [2]. The algorithm then optimally configures itself so that it cannot only provide the desired result when presented with the training inputs, but it can even generalize to produce the desired outcome from new data [2]. **Figure 3** shows a generic ML workflow. In which, the ML model is trained first on a training data then the trained model is used for predicting the results for new data [2]. More deeply, ML algorithms have been classified according to the nature of the data labeling into supervised (e.g., classification or regression), unsupervised (e.g., clustering and estimation of probability density function), and semi-supervised learning approach (e.g., text/image retrieval systems) [11–13].

With the era of big data, the utilization of machine learning algorithms in radiation oncology research is rapidly growing. Its applications include treatment response modeling, treatment planning, organ segmentation, image-guidance, motion tracking, quality assurance, and more. In this chapter, we provide the interested reader with an overview about the ongoing advances and cutting-edge applications of the ML methods in radiation oncology from a workflow perspective, from patient diagnosis and assessment to treatment delivery and follow-up. We present the areas where ML could be applied to improve the efficiency, i.e., optimizing and automating the clinical processes, and quality, i.e., potentials for decision-making support toward precision medicine in radiation therapy, of patient care. This chapter is organized as follows: Section 1 provides introduction to radiation oncology, big data, and machine learning concept; Section 2 illustrates an overview of the utilization of machine learning methods in radiation oncology research from a workflow perspective; Section 3 discusses limitations and the challenges of the of the current approaches as well as the future vision to overcome these problems; and Section 4 presents conclusions.

2. Machine learning in radiation oncology

The utilization of machine learning algorithms in radiation oncology research has covered almost every part in radiotherapy workflow process (**Figure 1**). ML techniques could compensate for human limitations in handling a large amount of flowing information in an efficient manner, in which simple errors can make the difference between life and death. Also, it would allow improvements in quality of patient care through the potentials toward a practical application of precision medicine in radiation oncology. In this section, we go over each part in the radiation oncology workflow (**Figure 1**) process presenting studies that have been conducted with machine learning models. The radiation oncology workflow starts with patient diagnosis and assessment, to treatment simulation, to treatment planning, to quality assurance and treatment delivery, to treatment outcome and follow-up.

2.1 Patient diagnosis, assessment, and consultation

The radiation oncology process begins at the first consultation. During which, the radiation oncologist and patient meet to discuss the clinical situation to determine a treatment strategy [14]. The stage that precedes the patient assessment and consultation is a patient diagnosis, in which patient with cancer disease identified on medical images and then pathologically confirmed the disease. Machine learning toolkits such as computer-aided detection/diagnosis have been introduced for identifying and classifying cancer subtypes (staging). For example, lesion candidates into abnormal or normal (identify and mark suspicious areas in an image), lesions or non-lesions (help radiologists decide if a patient should have a biopsy or not), malignant or benign (report the likelihood that a lesion is malignant), etc. Machine learning plays a crucial role in computer-aided detection/diagnosis toolkits, and it could provide a "second opinion" in decision-making to the physician in diagnostic radiology.

2.1.1 Computer-aided detection

Computer-aided detection (CADe) has defined as detection made by a physician/radiologist who takes into account the computer output as a "second opinion" [2]. CADe has been an active research area in medical imaging [2]. Its task is classification based solving a problem, in which the ML classifier task here is to determine "optimal" boundaries for separating classes in the multidimensional feature space. It focuses on a detection task, e.g., localization of lesions in medical images with the possibility of providing the likelihood of detection.

Several investigators [15–18] have developed ML-based models for detection of cancer, e.g., lung nodules [15] in thoracic computed tomography (CT) using massive training artificial neural network (ANN), micro-calcification breast masses [16] in mammography using a convolutional neural network (CNN), prostate cancer [17] and brain lesion [18] on magnetic resonance imaging (MRI) data using deep learning. Chan et al. [16] achieved a very good accuracy, an area under a receiver operating characteristic curve (AUC) of 0.90, in the automatic detection of clustered of breast microcalcifications on mammograms. Suzuki et al. [15] reported an improved accuracy in the detection of lung nodules in low-dose CT images. Zhu et al. [17] reported an averaged detection rate of 89.90% of prostate cancer on MR images, with clear indication that the high-level features learned from the deep learning method can achieve better performance than the handcrafted features in detecting prostate cancer regions. Rezaei et al. [18] results demonstrated the superior ability of the deep learning approach in brain lesions detection.

Overall, the use of computer-aided detection systems as a "second opinion" tool in identifying the lesion regions in the images would significantly contribute to improving diagnostic performance. For example, it would lead to avoid missing cancer regions, increase sensitivity and specificity of detection (increased accuracy), and diminish inter- and intraobserver variability.

2.1.2 Computer-aided diagnosis

Computer-aided diagnosis (CADx) is a computerized procedure to provide a "second objective opinion" for the assistance of medical image interpretation and diagnosis [19]. Similar to CADe, its task is a classification solving-problem. CADx focuses on a diagnosis (characterization) task, e.g., distinction and automatically classifying a tumor or lesion being malignant or benign with a possibility of providing the likelihood of diagnosis.

Numerous studies [19–22] have demonstrated the application of CADx tools for diagnosing lung [19–21] and breast [19, 22] lesions. Cheng et al. [19] investigated the deep learning capability for the diagnosis of breast lesions in ultrasound (US) images and pulmonary nodules in CT scans. Their results showed that the deep-learning-based CADx can achieve better differentiation performance than the comparison methods across different modalities and diseases. **Figure 4** illustrates several cases of breast lesions and pulmonary nodules in US and CT images, respectively, differentiated with deep learning-based CADx [19]. Feng et al. [20] and Beig et al. [21] studied the classification of lung lesions on endo-bronchoscopic images [20] with logistic regressions, and non-small cell lung cancer (NSCLC) adenocarcinomas distinctions from granulomas on non-contrast CT [21] using support vector machine (SVM) and neural network (NN). The reported results indicated an accuracy of 86% in distinguishing lung cancer types, e.g., adenocarcinoma and squamous cell carcinoma [20]. Surprisingly, the reported results [21] in distinguishing non-small cell lung cancer adenocarcinomas from granulomas on non-contrast CT images showed that the developed CADx systems outperformed the radiologist readers. Joo et al. [22] developed a CADx system using an ANN for breast nodule malignancy diagnosis in US images. Their results demonstrated the potential to increase the specificity of US for characterization of breast lesions.

Overall, computer-aided diagnosis tool as a "second opinion" system could significantly enhance the radiologists' performance by reducing the misdiagnosed rate of malignant cases, then decreases the false positive of the cases sent for surgical biopsy. Also with CADx, the diagnosis can be performed based on multimodality medical images in a non-invasive (without biopsy), fast (fast scanning) and a low-cost way (no additional examination cost).

2.1.3 Assessment and consultation

During the patient assessment phase, the radiation oncologist and patient meet to discuss the clinical situation. Circumstances like the risks and benefits of treatment and the patient's goals of care are determined for the treatment strategy [14]. Useful information to assess the potential benefit of treatment is acquired, e.g., tumor

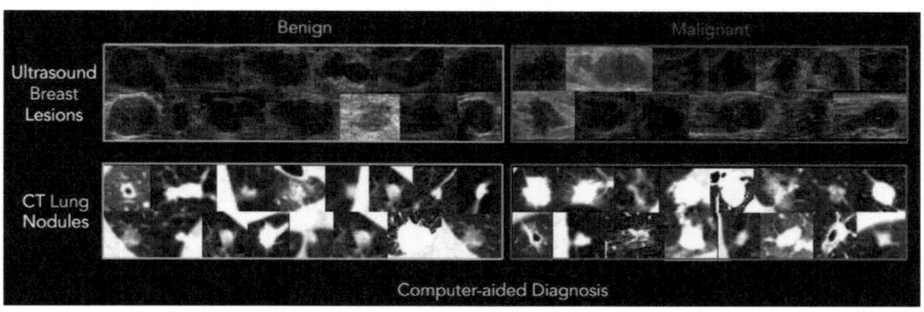

Figure 4.
Computer-aided diagnosis for lung nodules and breast lesion with deep learning. It shows that it may be hard to differentiate for a person without a medical background and for a junior medical doctor (reproduced from [19]).

stage, prior and current therapies, margin status if post-resection, ability to tolerate multimodality therapy, and overall performance status [14]. Parameters that impact potential risk and tolerability of treatment are balanced, e.g., patient age, comorbidities, functional status, the proximity between tumor and critical normal tissues, and ability to cooperate with motion management [14]. All of these represent valuable features which can be utilized to build predictive models of treatment outcome and toxicity. These models, then, can be used to inform physicians and patients to manage expectations and guide trade-offs between risks and benefit [14].

Machine learning models [23–26] such as logistic regressions, decision trees, random forests, gradient boosting, and support vector machines are suitable for this purpose. Logistic regressions or decision trees are similarly effective [23, 24] for a goal to assist physicians and patients reach the best decision, compromising balance between interpretability of the results and accurate predictions. In case of accuracy is favored over interpretability, then methods [25, 26] such as random forests or gradient boosting, and SVMs with kernels, are better and consistently win most modeling competitions [14].

Overall, the delivery of models that could help with these scenarios require standardizing nomenclature and developing standards for data collection of these heterogeneous patient clinical data remain a challenge in radiation oncology.

2.2 Treatment simulation

Once a physician and patient have decided to proceed with radiation therapy, the physician will place robust instructions for a simulation, which is then scheduled. The order for simulation includes details about immobilization, scan range, treatment site, and other specifics necessary to complete the procedure appropriately [14]. Patient preparation for simulation could include fiducial placement, fasting or bladder/rectal filling instructions, or kidney function testing for intravenous (IV) contrast. Special instructions have given for patients with a cardiac device, or who are pregnant, and lift help or a translator is requested if necessary [14]. The treatment simulation process typically includes patient's setup and immobilization, three- or four-dimensional computed tomography (3DCT or 4DCT) image data acquisition, and image reconstruction/segmentation. Machine learning algorithms could have an essential role to play in this sequence to improve the simulation quality, hence a better treatment outcome.

2.2.1 3D/4DCT image acquisition

Three-dimensional CT anatomical image information for the patient are acquired during the simulation on a dedicated CT scanner ("CT-Simulator") to be used later for the treatment planning purposes. A good CT simulation is critical to the success of all subsequent processes, to achieve an accurate, high quality, robust, and deliverable plan for a patient. It could prevent a repeated CT simulation due to insufficient scan range, suboptimal immobilization, non-optimal bladder/rectal filling, artifacts, lack of breath-hold reproducibility, and so on [14]. 4DCT scanning is used increasingly in radiotherapy departments to track the motion of tumors in relation to the respiratory cycle of the patient. It monitors the breathing cycle of the patient and can either; acquire CT images at a certain point in the breathing cycle, or acquire CT images over the whole breathing cycle. This CT data is then used to generate an ITV (internal target volume) that encompasses the motion of the CTV (clinical target volume), or MIP (maximum intensity projection) scans to aid in the definition of an ITV [2]. 4DCT imaging is necessary for successful implementation of stereotactic ablative radiotherapy (SBRT), e.g., for early-stage NSCLC.

Few works [27–30] have carried out using ML-based methods for this purpose. For instance, a work by Fayad et al. [27] demonstrated an ML method based on the principal component analysis (PCA) to develop a global respiratory motion model capable of relating external patient surface motion to internal structure motion without the need for a patient-specific 4DCT acquisition. Its finding looks promising but future works of assessing the model extensively are needed. Another study by Steiner et al. [28] investigated an ML-based model on correlations and linear regressions for quantifying whether 4DCT or 4D CBCT (cone-beam CT) represents the actual motion range during treatment using Calypso (Varian Medical Systems Inc., Palo Alto, CA, USA) motion signals as the "ground truth." The study results found that 4DCT and 4DCBCT under-predict intra-fraction lung target motion during radiotherapy. A third interesting one by Dick et al. [29] examined an ANN model for fiducial-less tracking for the radiotherapy of liver tumors through tracking lung-diaphragm border. The findings showed that the diaphragm and tracking volumes are closely related, and the method has indicated the potential to replace fiducial markers for clinical application. Finally, a study by Johansson et al. [30] investigated an ML-based PCA model for reconstructing breathing-compensated images showing the phases of gastrointestinal (GI) motion. Its results indicated that GI 4D MRIs could help define internal target volumes for treatment planning or support GI motion tracking during irradiation.

Overall, the discussed ML-based methods in the simulation area have shown the potential for improved accuracy of patient CT simulation. Machine learning utilization in 3D/4D CT image acquisition simulation is an area where the community has focused little effort. Thus, focusing on the simulation, there are many questions that could be answered/optimized through ML algorithms to aid in decision-making and overall workflow efficiency.

2.2.2 Image reconstruction

Here, we explore the power of machine learning based methods for image reconstruction in radiation oncology procedure. We present two application examples where ML has utilized for estimating CT from MRI images and reconstructing a 7 Tesla (7 T)-like MR image from a 3 T MR image.

The first application supports reconstructing an image modality form another imaging modality, e.g., CT image from MR image. Clinical implementation of MRI-only treatment planning radiotherapy approach requires a method to derive or reconstruct synthetic CT image from MR image. CT is currently supporting the workflows of radiation oncology treatment planning for dose calculations. However, CT imaging modality has some limitations in comparison with other modalities like MRI, e.g., (a) CT images provide poor soft tissue contrast compared to MRI scans which has superior visualization of anatomical structures and tumors, and (b) CT exposes radiation during CT imaging, which may cause side effect to the patient, where MRI is much safer and does not involve radiation.

Numerous studies [31–34] have demonstrated ML-based approaches to map CT images to MR images like deep learning (fully CNN) model [31], boosting-based sampling (RUSBoost) algorithm [32], random forest and auto-context model [33], and U-net CNN model [34]. Nie et al. [31] experimental results showed that deep learning method is accurate and robust for predicting CT image from MRI image. **Figure 5** shows the synthetic CT image from MRI data with deep learning and the "ground truth" MRI [31]. The developed deep learning model outperformed other state-of-the-art methods under comparison. Bayisa et al. [32] proposed an approach based on boosting algorithm indicated outperformance in CT estimation quality in comparison with the existing model-based methods on the brain and bone tissues.

Huynh et al. [33] experimental results showed that a structured random forest and auto-context based model can accurately predict CT images in various scenarios, and also outperformed two state-of-the-art methods. Chen et al. [34] investigated the feasibility of a deep CNN for MRI-based synthetic CT generation. The gamma analysis of their results with "ground truth" CT image for 1%/1 mm gamma pass rates was over 98.03%. The dosimetric accuracy on the dose-volume histogram (DVH) parameters discrepancy was less than 0.87% and the maximum point dose discrepancy within PTV (planning target volume) was less than 1.01% respect to the prescription on prostate intensity modulated radiotherapy (IMRT) planning.

Overall, the presented findings have obviously demonstrated the potential of the discussed methods to generate synthetic CT images to support the MR-only workflow of radiotherapy treatment planning and image guidance.

The second application supports reconstructing a high-quality image modality from a lower quality one, e.g., 7 T-like MR image from 3 T MR image. The advanced ultra—high 7 T magnetic field scanners provide MR images with higher resolution and better tissue contrast compared to routine 3 T MRI scanners. However, 7 T MRI scanners are currently more expensive, less available in clinical centers, and higher restrictions are required for safety due to its extremely high magnetic field power. As a result, generating/reconstructing a 7 T-like MR image from a 3 T MR image with ML-based approaches would resolve these concerns as well as facilitate early disease diagnosis.

Researchers [35–38] have developed ML-based models to generate a 7 T-like MR image from 3 T MR image. Approaches based on deep learning CNN [35], hierarchical reconstruction based on group sparsity in a novel multi-level canonical correlation analysis (CCA) space [36], and random forest and sparse representation [37, 38] have been investigated to map 3 T MR images to be as 7 T-like MR images. Bahrami et al. [35] visual and numerical results showed that deep learning method outperformed the comparison methods. **Figure 6** presents the reconstruction of 7 T-like MR image from 3 T MR image with deep learning. A second study [36] done by the same author showed that a hierarchical reconstruction based on group sparsity method outperformed other previous methods and resulted in higher accuracy in the segmentation of brain structures, compared to segmentation of 3 T MR images. Other studies by Bahrami et al. [37, 38] using random forest regression model and a group sparse representation showed that the predicted 7 T-like MR images can best match the "ground-truth" 7 T MR images, compared to other methods. Moreover, the experiment on brain tissue segmentation showed that predicted 7 T-like MR images lead to the highest accuracy in the segmentation, compared to segmentation of 3 T MR images.

Overall, the predicted 7 T-like MR images have demonstrated better spatial resolution compared to 3 T MR images. Moreover, delineation critical structure,

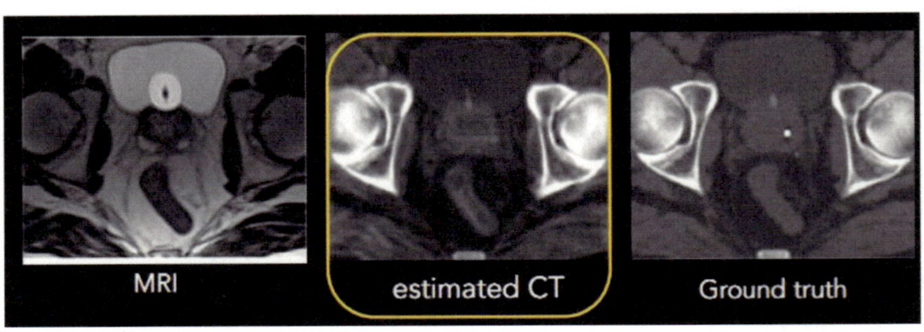

Figure 5.
Synthetic CT image from MRI data. MR image (left), estimated CT form the MR (middle) with deep learning, and "ground truth" (right) MR image for the same subject (reproduced from [31]).

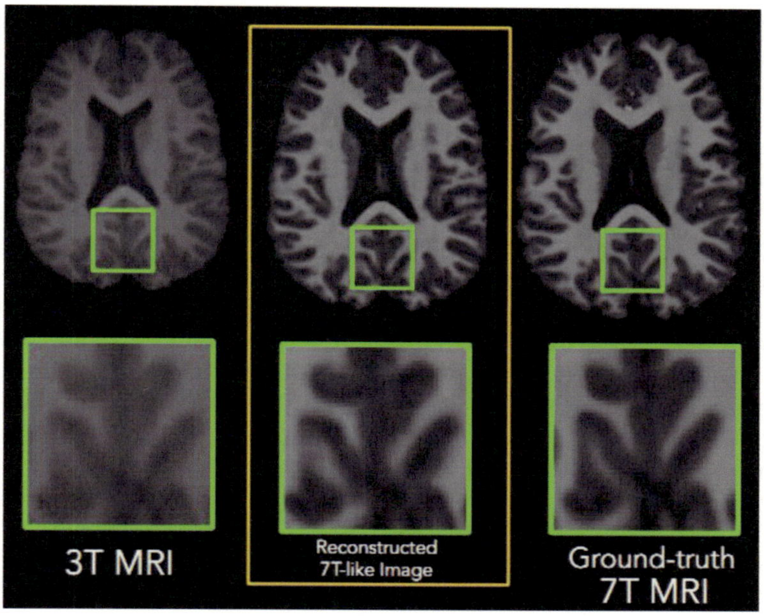

Figure 6.
Reconstruction of 7 T-like MR image from 3 T MR image. 3 T MR image (left), reconstructed 7 T-like MR image (middle) using deep learning, and 7 T MR "ground truth" image (left) of the same subject with each one corresponded with a same selected zoomed area. From the figure, 7 T MR image shows clearly better anatomical details and tissue contrast compared to 3 T MR image (reproduced from [35]).

i.e., brain tissue structures on 7 T-like MR images showed better accuracy compared to segmentation of 3 T MR images. Adding to above, such high-quality 7 T-like MR image could better help disease diagnosis and intervention.

2.2.3 Image registration/fusion

Image registration in radiotherapy is the process of aligning images rigidly which allows some changes in images to be easily detected. However, such an alignment does not model changes from, e.g., organ deformation, patient weight loss, or tumor shrinkage. It is possible to take such changes into account using deformable image registration (DIR) which is a method for finding the mapping between points in one image and the corresponding points in another image. DIR has the perspective of being widely integrated into many different steps of the radiotherapy process. The tasks of planning, delivery, and evaluation of radiotherapy can all be improved by taking organ deformation into account. Use of image registration in image-guided radiotherapy (IGRT) can be split into intra-patient (*inter- and intra-fractionated*) and inter-patient registration. Intra-patient registration is matching of images of a single patient, e.g., *inter-fractional registration* (i.e., improving patient positioning, and evaluating organ motion relative to bones) and *intra-fractional registration* (i.e., online tracking of organ movement). In contrast, inter-patient registration is matching images from different patients (i.e., an "average" of images acquired from a number of patients, thereby allowing information to be transferred from the atlas to the newly acquired image). The process of combining information from two images after these have been registered is called data fusion. A particular use of data transfer between images is the propagation of contours from the planning image or an atlas to a newly acquired image [39, 40]. Although many image registration methods have been proposed, there are still some challenges for DIR of complex situations, e.g., large anatomical changes and dynamic appearance changes.

Advancement in computer vision and deep learning could provide solutions to overcome these challenges of conventional rigid/deformable image registrations.

Various machine learning-based methods [41–47] for image registration have proposed by investigators to not only align the anatomical structures but also alleviate the appearance difference. Hu et al. [41] proposed a method based on regression forest for image registration of two arbitrary MR images. The learning-based registration method achieved higher registration accuracy compared with other counterpart registration methods. Zagoruyko et al. [42] proposed a general similarity function for comparing image patches, which is a task for many computer vision problems. The results showed that such an approach like CNN-based model can significantly outperform other state-of-the-art methods. Jiang et al. [43] employed a discriminative local derivative pattern method to achieve fast and robust multimodal image registration. The results revealed that the proposed method can achieve superior performance regarding accuracy in multimodal image registration as well as also indicated the potential for clinical US-guided intervention. Neylon et al. [44] developed a deep neural network for automated quantification of DIR performance. Their results showed a correlation between the NN predicted error and the "ground truth" for the PTV and the organs at risk (OARs) were consistently observed to be greater than 0.90. Wu et al. [45, 46] developed an NN-based registration quality evaluator, and a deep learning-based image registration framework, respectively, to improve the image registration robustness. The quality evaluator method [45] showed potentials to be used in a 2D/3D rigid image registration system to improve the overall robustness, and the new image registration framework [46] consistently demonstrated more accurate registration results when compared to the state-of-the-art. Kearney et al. [47] developed a deep unsupervised learning strategy for CBCT to CT deformable image registration. The results indicated that deep learning method performed better than rigid registration, intensity corrected demons and landmark-guided deformable image registration for all evaluation metrics.

Overall, most of the machine learning based methods discussed here for image registration have revealed superior performance regarding accuracy in multimodal image registration. Hence, potentials for improved rigid/deformable image registration in radiation oncology are clinically feasible.

2.2.4 Image segmentation/auto-contouring

Volume definition is a prerequisite for meaningful 3D treatment planning and for accurate dose reporting. International Commission on Radiation Units and Measurements (ICRU) Reports No. 50, 62, 71 and 83 [48] define and describe target volumes (e.g., planning target volume) and critical structure/normal tissue (organ at risk) volumes that aid in the treatment planning process and that provide a basis for comparison of treatment outcomes. The organ at risk is an organ whose sensitivity to radiation is such that the dose received from a treatment plan may be significant compared with its tolerance, possibly needs to be delineated to evaluate its received dose [49]. Multimodal diagnostic images, e.g., CT, MRI, US, positron emission tomography (PET)/CT, etc. can be used through image fusion to help in the process of delineating tumor and OAR structures on CT slices acquired during the patient's treatment simulation. The delineation (auto-contouring) process has subsequently become performed via automated or semi-automated analytical model-based software commercially available for clinical use (e.g., Atlas based-models). These software tools are performing reasonably well for critical organs/OARs delineation but not yet ready for tumor/target structures contouring which represent a challenging task. State-of-the-art machine learning algorithms may play an effective role here for both tasks.

Several ML-based methods [52–58] have reported for tumor/target segmentation/auto-contouring, e.g., brain [52–55], prostate [56], rectum [57], sclerosis lesion [58], etc. The reported results showed that deep learning [54, 55] and ensemble learning [50, 53] ML-based methods are the winner algorithms over the other ML-based methods in the brain tumor segmentation competitions [50]. Such a method by Osman [52] based on SVM for glioma brain tumor segmentation showed a robust consistency performance on the training and new "unseen" testing data even though its reported accuracy on multi-institution datasets was reasonably acceptable. **Figure 7** shows the whole glioma brain tumor segmentation on MRI (BRATS'2017 dataset [50, 51]) with an SVM model [52]. For organs segmentation, deep learning algorithm [57, 59, 60] has shown a superior performance than other state-of-the-art segmentation methods and commercially available software for segmentation of, e.g., rectum [57], parotid [59], etc.

Overall, tumor/target segmentation/auto-contouring using ML-based methods still remains challenging for some reasons such as availability of big data of multi-modal images with their "ground truth" annotation data for training these models. Recent advances in computer vision, specifically around deep learning [61], are particularly well suited for segmentation and it has shown superiority over the other machine learning algorithms for tumor and organs segmentation tasks.

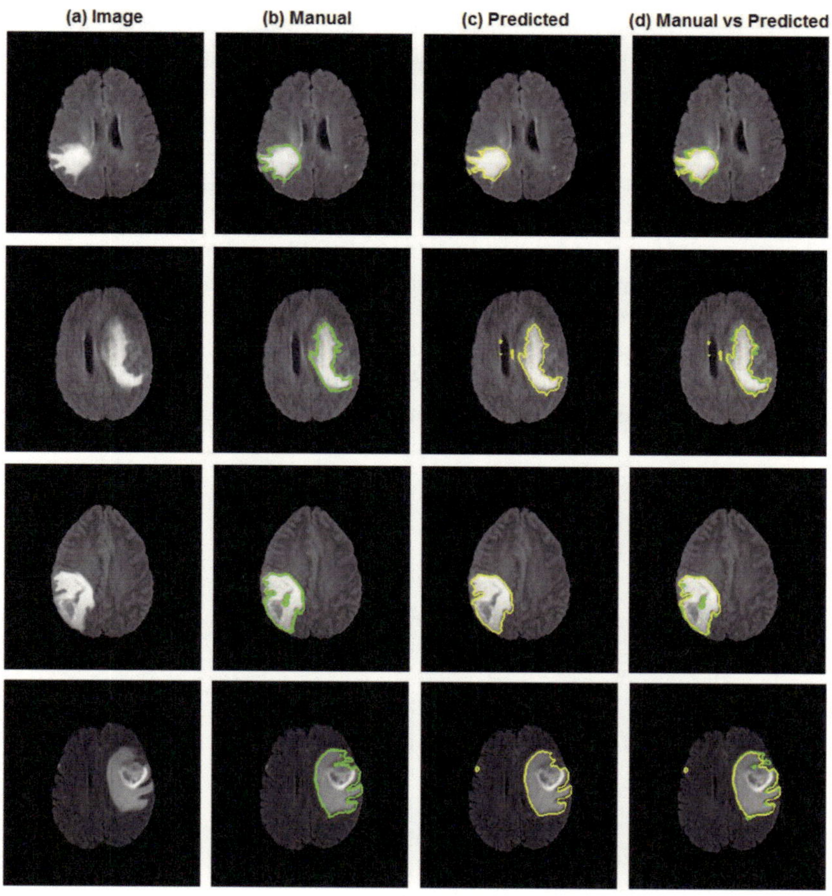

Figure 7.
Whole glioma brain tumor segmentation on MRI (BRATS'2017 dataset [50, 51]). (a) T2-FLAIR MRI, (b) manual "ground truth" glioma segmentation by an experienced board-certified radiation oncologist, (c) machine learning—SVM model glioma segmentation [52], and (d) both, manual and ML, segmented annotations overlap; for four different subjects.

2.3 Treatment planning

The planning process starts by delineating both the target(s) and the OARs as we discussed it earlier in the image segmentation section (Section 2.2.4). Once the target volumes and OARs have been outlined/contoured, the planning process continues by (1) setting dosimetric goals for targets and normal tissues; (2) selecting an appropriate treatment technique (e.g., 3D, fixed beam IMRT, VMAT (volumetric arc radiation therapy), protons); (3) iteratively modifying the beams/weights/etc., until the planning goals have been achieved; and (4) evaluating (estimating the treatment dose distributions with prescribed doses in the treatment planning system using dose calculation algorithms) and approving the plan [14]. The applications of machine learning in radiotherapy treatment planning as a tool for knowledge-based treatment planning (KBTP) and automated/self-driven planning process will be discussed in this section.

2.3.1 Knowledge-based treatment planning

Prior information about patient status and previously archived treatment plans, particularly if performed by expert medical dosimetrists/physicists, could be used to inform the treating team of a currently pending case [2]. This concept of using prior treatment planning information constitutes the underlying principle of the so-called knowledge-based treatment planning. Such KBTP approaches have leveraged hundreds of prior treatment plans to reproducibly improve planning efficiency across multiple disease sites [62]. **Figure 8** illustrates the schematic of a KBTP System [2]. The motivation for KBTP approach lies in reducing current complexity and time spent on generating a new treatment plan from each incoming patient, as well as its potential for decision-making support in radiotherapy.

Several studies [63–67] have carried out to explore the utilization of KBTP approach for treatment plan generation in radiotherapy. The current scientific research and available commercial products for KBTP are limited to predicting DVHs within accepted ranges [14]. Plans generated based on KBTP utilizing artificial intelligence often meet or exceed adherence to dose constraints compared to manually generated plans in many clinical scenarios (e.g., prostate cancer [63], cervical cancer [64], gliomas and meningiomas [65], head and neck cancer [66], and spine SBRT [67]). A more recent commercial product, Quick Match

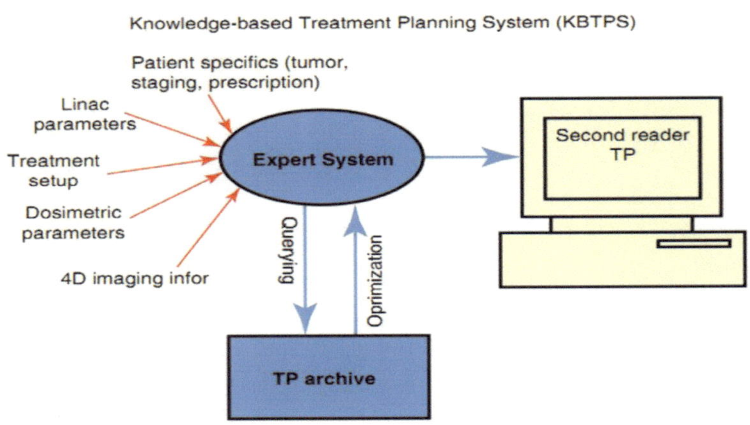

Figure 8.
Schematic of a KBTP system. Initially, the user builds a query using features related to patient, disease, imaging, treatment setup, dose, etc., for the treatment plan (TP). Then, the database returns a set of similar treatment plans that the user could select from to optimize and compare with the current one according to the query (reproduced from [2]).

(Siris Medical, Redwood City, CA, USA), uses gradient boosting (the most accurate algorithm on expectation when structured data are available) to explore predictions in dosimetric trade-offs [68]. This application provides quick rough predicted treatment planning results to be obtained before the treatment planning process. Thus it can facilitate communication between dosimetrist and physicians, establish individualized and achievable goals, and help physicians and patients decide the course of a plan before initializing the treatment planning process. For example, it can help to choose an optimal technique (e.g., photon versus protons). This approach has also been applied to post-planning quality assurance of DVH data [69, 70].

Overall, the incentive for such an approach like KBTP lies in reducing current complexity and time spent on generating a new treatment plan from each incoming patient. It is believed that such a standardization process based on KBTP can help enhance consistency, efficiency, and plan quality. Ultimately, data-driven planning is not fully automated at present as it requires expert oversight and/or intervention to ensure safely deliverable treatment plans.

2.3.2 Automated planning (self-driving) process

Once the dosimetric goals have been established and the technique chosen, automatic plan generation is also possible [14].

Some attempts [71, 72] have made to solve various aspects of this problem by predicting the best beam orientations. The larger task of automated treatment planning, however, is well suited for reinforcement learning method [14]. Reinforcement is extensively used in games, self-driving cars, and other popular-culture applications. In reinforcement learning method, an algorithm learns to navigate a set of rules, given some constraints, by self-correcting its decisions. Basically, the algorithm will take a decision (for instance, increase the weight of a given constraint) and learn from the simulator (the treatment planning system) whether the decision resulted in the right direction [14]. This technique has successfully used by Google Brain to develop an algorithm capable of beating a Go world champion [73]. So, reinforcement technique could provide performance at the level of our best dosimetrists if properly implemented.

Overall, one challenge of achieving full automatic planning using reinforcement learning lies in the close integration and need for robust treatment planning systems (TPSs) [14]. The future vision is toward a fully-automated planning process, from contouring to plan creation [62], with the human experts (dosimetrists, physicists, and physicians) evaluating, supervising, and providing QA to the given results.

2.4 Quality assurance and treatment delivery

Quality assurance (QA) is demanding for the safe delivery of radiotherapy. It represents a core part of a medical physicist's task in the clinical practice. Machine learning could be utilized to solve multiple long-standing problems and improve workflow efficiency. Its applications in the quality assurance (e.g., detection and prediction of radiotherapy errors, and treatment planning QA) and treatment delivery validation (e.g., prediction planning deviations from the initial intentions, and prediction the need for re-planning for adaptive radiotherapy) are discussed in this section.

2.4.1 Quality assurance

Machine learning has potential in many aspects of radiotherapy QA program, specifically in error detection and prevention, treatment machine QA, patient-specific quality assurance, etc. In addition, ML may contribute to automating the

QA process and analysis, which significantly influence an increase in efficiency and a decrease in the physical effort in performing the QA.

Numerous studies [74–77, 79–83] have conducted to develop a computerized system for QA process based on machine learning methods. We can generally categorize these QA into the machine-based and patient-based approach. For machine-based QA approach, ML utilizations for automatic QA process of medical linear accelerator (Linac) machine [74–77] have investigated by research scientists. A study by Li et al. [74] investigated the application of ANN to monitor the performance of the Linac for continuous improvement of patient safety and quality of care. The preliminary results showed better accuracy and effective applicability in the dosimetry and QA field over other techniques, and in some cases, its performance beat the detection rate by current clinical metrics. El Naqa et al. [75] introduced a system utilizing anomaly detection to overcome the problem of direct modeling of QA errors and rare events in radiotherapy and to support the intent of automated QA and safety management for patients undergo radiotherapy treatment. Ford et al. [76] and Hoisak et al. [77] investigated quantifying the error-detection effectiveness of commonly used quality control (QC) measures [76] preventative maintenance [77] in radiation oncology. The results indicated that the effectiveness of QC measures in radiation oncology depends sensitively on which checks are used and in which combinations [76], and also a decreased machine downtime and other technical failures leading to treatment cancellations [77]. The ability of these ML algorithms to automatically detect outliers allows physicists to focus attention on those aspects of a process most likely to impact the patient care, as recommended in AAPM Task Group report 100 [78].

For patient-based QA approach, application of ML algorithms for a plan and patient-specific QA, multi-leaf collimators (MLCs) QA, and imaging [79–83] have discovered by many investigators. A study by Valdes et al. [80] investigated the use of SVM-based system to automatically detect problems with the Linac 2D/3D imaging system that are used for patient IGRT treatment accuracy. The proposed method results showed that the bare minimum and the best practice QA programs could be implemented with the same manpower. Regarding plan QA and patient-specific QA, investigators [81, 82] studied applications of Poisson regression with LASSO regularization to predict individualized IMRT QA passing rates. Their results pointed out that virtual IMRT QA can predict passing rates with a high likelihood, allows the detection of failures due to setup errors. Osman et al. [79] and Carlson et al. [83] utilized NN and a cubist algorithm, respectively, to predict MLC positional errors using the Linac generated log file data of IMRT and VMAT delivered plans. Their studies results showed that predicted parameters were in closer agreement to the delivered parameters than the planned parameters. The inclusion of these predicted deviations in leaves positioning into the TPS during dose calculation leads to a more realistic representation of plan delivery. **Figure 9** illustrates a generic flow diagram and results of an NN utilized for prediction of MLCs positional errors [79].

Overall, despite these significant improvements in QA processes with the involvement of ML, they carry implicit maintenance costs in the form of additional QA demands for the algorithms themselves. The performance of all deployed ML-based algorithms will, therefore, need to be verified periodically using an evolving series of tests [62]. Virtual QA can have profound implications on the current IMRT/VMAT process and potentially enabling intelligent resource allocation in favor of plans more likely to fail.

2.4.2 Treatment delivery

Tumor shrinkage and anatomical patient variations (e.g., due to weight loss) may occur throughout a few weeks of a fractionated radiotherapy treatment. Adaptive

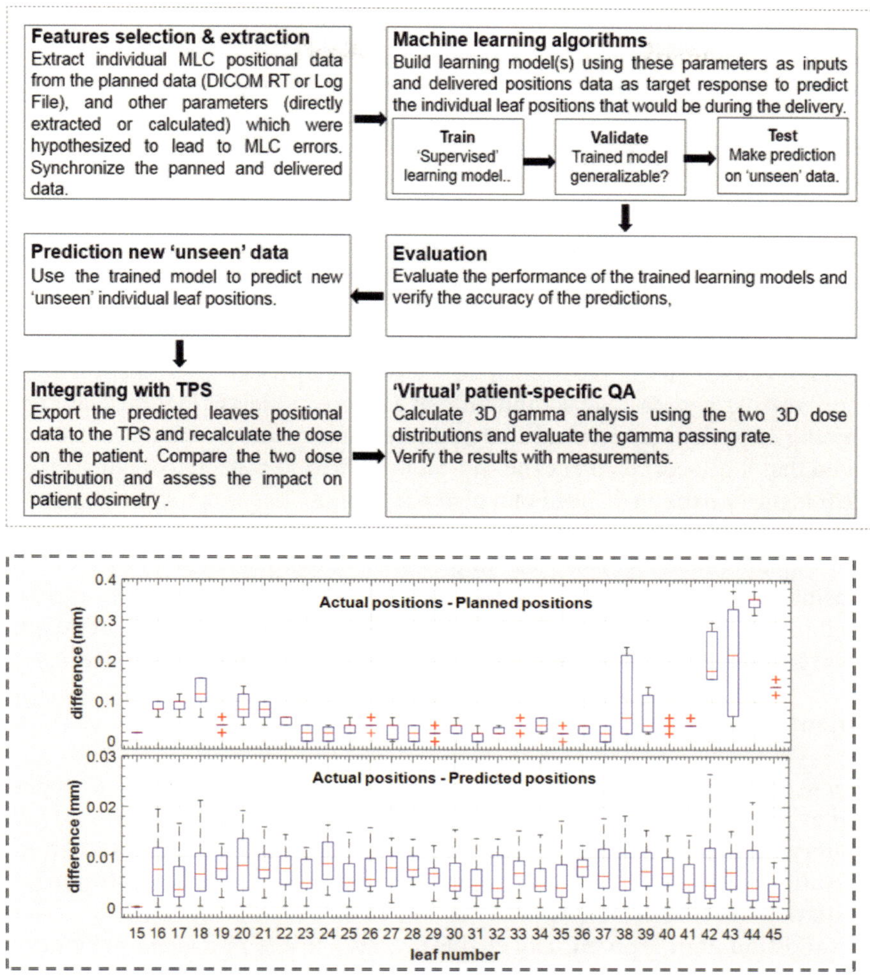

Figure 9.
Top: A generic flow diagram of the proposed method of prediction MLC positional errors [79]. Bottom: Differences in the leaf positions between the delivered and planned (upper), and delivered and predicted with NN (lower). Boxes report quartiles including the median (the 50% central sample distribution); whiskers and dots indicate outliers.

radiation therapy (ART) is a treatment approach that uses frequent imaging to compensate for anatomical differences that occur during the course of treatment. Images are taken daily, or almost daily. When significant changes are observed, replanning is considered. It is possible to achieve image-guided adaptation either off-line (i.e., using image information acquired during a fraction for improving following fraction) or online (i.e., changing treatment plan for a fraction based on information from the same fraction).

The re-planning process involves three steps [84]: (1) simulating the plan from the daily CBCT image dataset to calculate the estimated actual delivered daily dose for the given treatment fraction, (2) delineating the structures of interest to obtain daily DVHs to provide dose metrics for the tumor and OARs from which radiation oncologists can evaluate treatment plan effectiveness, and (3) modifying the doses to the therapeutic target and OARs to meet the dose constraints in the original treatment plan. The implementation of adaptive radiotherapy into routine clinical practice is technically challenging and requires significant resources to perform and validate each process step. It needs to be fast (where time is a big issue) in order to fit into the clinical workflow. Machine learning techniques, i.e., deep learning, may offer potentials to have very sophisticated software tools for adaptive therapy. In recent years, deep learning [61] applications have grown in a variety of fields including video games, computer vision, and pattern recognition.

A number of researchers [85–88] have investigated the application of ML, particularly deep learning, in treatment re-planning process for adaptive radiotherapy. Studies by Guidi et al. [85] and Chetvertkov et al. [86] conducted to predict patients who would benefit from ART and re-planning intervention using SVM [85] and PCA [86] ML models. The studies results indicated a capability of identifying patients would benefit from ART and ideal time for a re-planning intervention. Tseng et al. [87] investigated deep reinforcement learning based on historical treatment plans for developing automated radiation adaptation protocols for lung cancer patients aiming to maximize tumor local control at reduced rates of radiation pneumonitis. The study findings revealed that automated dose adaptation by deep reinforcement learning is a feasible and promising approach for achieving similar results to those chosen by clinicians. Varfalvy et al. [88] introduced a new automated patient classification method based on relative gamma analysis and hidden Markov models to identify patients undergoing important anatomical changes during radiotherapy. The results obtained indicated that it can complement the clinical information collected during treatment and help identify patients in need of a plan adaptation.

Overall, adaptive radiotherapy demands a high-speed planning system, combined with high-quality imaging. Deep learning-based ML methods have shown potential and feasibility to transform adaptive radiation therapy more effectively and efficiently into the routine clinical practice soon. Effective implementation of adaptive radiation therapy can further improve the precision in the radiotherapy treatments.

2.5 Patient follow-up

Patient follow-up begins at the start of the treatment and continues to beyond the end of the treatment. Accurate prediction of treatment outcomes would provide clinicians with better tools for informed decision-making about expected benefits versus anticipated risks [2]. Machine learning has the potential to revolutionize the way radiation oncologists follow patients treated with definitive radiation therapy [14]. In addition, it may potentially enable practical use of precision medicine in radiation oncology by predicting treatment outcomes for individual patients using radiomics "tumor/healthy tissue phenotypes" analysis.

2.5.1 Treatment outcome

Radiotherapy treatment outcomes are determined by complex interactions among treatment, anatomical, and patient-related variables [2]. A key component of radiation oncology research is to predict at the time of treatment planning, or during the course of fractionated radiation treatment, the tumor control probability (TCP) and normal tissue control probability (NTCP) for the type of treatment being considered for that particular patient [2]. Recent approaches have utilized increasingly data-driven models incorporating advanced bioinformatics and machine learning tools in which dose-volume metrics are mixed with other patients- or disease-based prognostic factors in order to improve outcomes prediction [2]. Obviously, better models based on early assessment are needed to predict the outcome, in time for treatment intensification with additional radiotherapy, early addition of systemic therapy, or application of a different treatment modality [14].

Many research scientists [89–95] have investigated the application of ML in radiotherapy treatment response and outcome predictions. Lee et al. [89] studied utilizing of Bayesian network ensemble to predict radiation pneumonitis risk for NSCLC patients whom received curative 3D conformal radiotherapy. The preliminary results demonstrated that such framework combined with an ensemble method can possibly improve the prediction of radiation pneumonitis under real-life clinical circumstances.

Naqa et al. [90] introduced a data mining framework estimating model parameters for predicting TCP using statistical resampling and a logistic, SVM, logistic regression, Poisson-based TCP, and cell kill equivalent uniform dose model. Their findings indicated that prediction of treatment response can be improved by utilizing data mining approaches, which were able to unravel important non-linear complex interactions among model variables and have the capacity to predict on unseen data for prospective clinical applications. Zhen et al. [91] introduced a CNN model to analyze the rectum dose distribution and predict rectum toxicity. The evaluation results demonstrated the feasibility of building a CNN-based rectum dose-toxicity prediction model with transfer learning for cervical cancer radiotherapy. Deist et al. [92] studied the comparison of six ML classifiers (namely, decision tree, random forest, NN, SVM, elastic net logistic regression, and LogitBoost) for chemo-radiotherapy to estimate their average discriminative performance for radiation treatment outcome prediction. The study results indicated that random forest and elastic net logistic regression yield higher discriminative performance in (chemo) radiotherapy outcome and toxicity prediction than other studied classifiers. Yahya et al. [93] explored multiple statistical-learning strategies for prediction of urinary symptoms following external beam radiotherapy of the prostate. The study results showed that logistic regression and multivariate adaptive regression splines (MARS) were most likely to be the best-performing strategy for the prediction of urinary symptoms. Zhang et al. [94] studied the prediction of organ-at-risk complications as a function of dose-volume constraint settings using SVMs and decisions trees. Their results showed that ML can be used for predicting OAR complications during treatment planning allowing for alternative dose-volume constraint settings to be assessed within the IMRT planning framework. A review by Kang et al. [95] presented the use of ML to predict radiation therapy outcomes from the clinician's point of view. The study focused on three popular ML methods: logistic regression, SVM, and ANN. The study concluded that although current studies are in exploratory stages, the overall methodology has progressively matured, and the field is ready for larger-scale further investigation.

Overall, a significant hope of advanced clinical informatics systems would be the potential to learn even more about the safety and effectiveness of the therapies that are provided to patients. The rapid adoption of technological advancements in radiotherapy has made outcomes analyses of both treatment regimens and the systems that deliver them to be separated substantially in time. Successful application of advanced ML tools for radiation oncology big data is essential to better-predicting radiotherapy treatment response and outcomes. The ultimate measure of success is an improvement in outcomes which can manifest as decreased toxicity or increased tumor control.

2.5.2 Radiomics for "precision medicine" radiotherapy

Precision medicine is a treatment strategy for making decisions about a molecularly targeted agent according to genetic mutations, rather than affected organs. Radiomics is the comprehensive quantitative analysis of medical images in order to extract a large number of phenotypic features (including those based on size and shape, image intensity, texture, relationships between voxels, and fractal characteristics) reflecting cancer traits or phenotypes. Then it explores the associations between the features and patients' prognoses in order to improve decision-making at each radiation treatment step (diagnosis, treatment planning, treatment delivery, and follow-up) and hence precision medicine in radiotherapy [96]. Individual patients can be stratified into subtypes based on radiomic biomarkers that contain information about cancer traits that determine the patient's prognosis [97]. Machine-learning algorithms can then be deployed to correlate the computer-extracted image-based features in radiomics with biological observations or clinical outcomes. Here, we present some current results and emerging paradigms in radiomics boosted with ML approaches in clinical radiation oncology (recently received higher attention from the investigators) to maximize its potential impact on precision radiotherapy.

Several research scientists [97–102] have investigated the using of ML methods for predicting radiotherapy outcomes (e.g., survival, treatment failure or recurrence, toxicity or developed a late complication, etc.) using radiomics features to improve decision-making for precision medicine. A review study by Arimura et al. [97] showed that radiomic approaches in combination with AI may potentially enable the practical use of precision medicine in radiation therapy by predicting outcomes and toxicity for individual patients. Aerts et al. [98] performed a radiomic analysis of 440 features quantifying tumor image intensity, shape, and texture, which are extracted from CT data of patients with lung or head-and-neck cancer. The study findings proved the power of radiomics for identifying a general prognostic phenotype existing in both lung and head-and-neck cancer. **Figure 10** shows a workflow of radiomics analysis (example: CT radiomic analysis of with lung cancer) [98]. A study by Depeursinge et al. [99] investigated the importance of pre-surgical CT intensity and texture information from ground-glass opacities and solid nodule components for the prediction of adenocarcinoma recurrence in the lung using LASSO and SVMs, and their survival counterparts: Cox-LASSO and survival SVMs. The study results showed the usefulness of the method in clinical practice to identify patients for which no recurrence is expected with very high confidence using a pre-surgical CT scan only. Lambin et al. [100] studied the development of automated and reproducible analysis methodologies to extract more information from image-based features. The study addressed the radiomics as one of the approaches that hold great promises but need further validation in multi-centric settings. A review by Wu et al. [101] recommended that ultimately prospective validation in multi-center clinical trials will be needed to demonstrate the clinical validity and utility of newly identified imaging markers and truly establish the value of radiomics and radiogenomics in precision radiotherapy. Lao et al. [102] investigated if deep features extracted via transfer learning can generate radiomics signatures for prediction of overall survival in patients with glioblastoma multiforme using the LASSO Cox regression model. The study outcomes demonstrated that the proposed method is capable to generate prognostic imaging signature for OS prediction

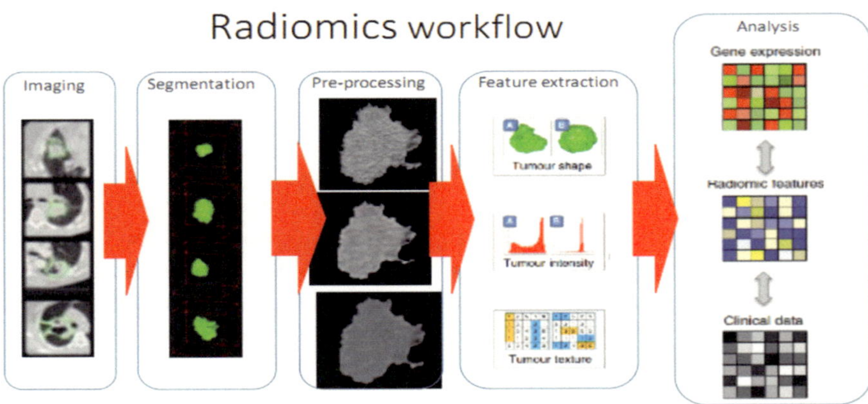

Figure 10.
A typical radiomics workflow. Imaging: Tumors are different. Example CT images with tumor contours of lung cancer patients. Segmentation: 3D visualizations of tumor contours delineated by experienced physicians on all CT slices. Pre-processing: Strategy for extracting radiomics data from images. Feature Extraction: Features are extracted from the defined tumor contours on the CT images quantifying tumor intensity, shape, texture and wavelet texture. Analysis: For the analysis, the radiomics features are compared with clinical data and gene-expression data (reproduced from [98]).

and patient stratification for glioblastoma, indicating the potential of deep imaging feature-based biomarker in preoperative care of glioblastoma patients.

Overall, radiomics is the study of imaging data from any imaging source that is used to predict the therapeutic outcome, as well as radiogenomics. The limited reproducibility of imaging systems both within and across institutions remains a significant challenge for radiomics [98, 100]. Application of deep learning to image quantification has produced stellar results in other areas [103] which can be transferred into the radiomics analysis. Physicians may prescribe a more or less intense radiation regimen for an individual based on model predictions of local control benefit and toxicity risk [2], which would be considered for the optimal treatment planning design process and hence improving the quality of life for radiotherapy cancer patients. Also, as imaging is routinely used in clinical practice, radiomics is providing an unprecedented opportunity to improve decision-making support toward precision medicine in cancer treatment at low cost.

3. Discussion

A comprehensive review of the most recent evolution and ongoing research utilizing machine learning methods in radiation oncology in the era of big data for precision medicine has been provided in this chapter and critically discussed.

3.1 Big data in radiation oncology: challenges?

There are ongoing community-wide efforts in term of big data in radiation oncology, e.g., [9, 10, 50, 51] have made available and established validation frameworks [50] used as a benchmark for the evaluation of different algorithms. Deep learning [61] based models have indicated superiority among the other alternatives for the most prediction tasks in radiation oncology. However, it requires a lot of annotated datasets (across multiple institutions) to tune the algorithm (even when transfer learning is used [14]) to obtain high prediction accuracy. This can prove challenging in radiation oncology, where datasets are limited. Standardizing the radiation oncology nomenclature (i.e., clinical, dosimetric, imaging, etc.), which is aided by the AAPM task group TG-263 efforts [104], and developing standards for data collection process (structures) of the patient data are also essential for training models using datasets from multiple institutions.

3.2 What are the strengths and limitations of ML algorithms applied?

There is no one algorithm works best for every problem ("No Free Lunch"). Each ML algorithm has its strengths and limitations. **Table 1** lists the strengths and weaknesses of the most machine learning methods discussed here appearing in radiation oncology studies. It is believed that such usage optimization of these models with available resources would provide improved solutions. A major limitation in the acceptance of ML by the larger medical community has been addressed as the "black box" stigma, where the ML algorithm maps a given input data to output predictions without providing any additional insight into the system mapping [6]. Interpretability of algorithms used (e.g., the ability for humans experts to understand the reasons behind a prediction) will play an important role to avoid preventable errors. Although there are inherently interpretable ML algorithms, for instance, decision trees, Bayesian networks, or generalized linear models (e.g., logistic regression), they are usually outperformed in terms of accuracy by ensemble methods or deep neural networks (not interpretable and provide very

Method	Strengths	Weaknesses
Decision tree	Interpretability (with a format consistent with many clinical pathways)	Overgrowing a tree with too few observations at leaf nodes
Random forest	Often can produce very accurate predictions with little feature engineering	Not easily interpretable, and not optimizing the number of trees
LASSO regression	Better interpretability (compared to ridge regularization method)	Provides a bias towards zero (not be appropriate in some applications)
Gradient boosting machines	Generates very stable results (compared to random forest)	More tuning parameters (compared to random forest), and overfitting
Support vector machines	Very accurate, few parameters that require tuning, and kernels options	Not readily interpretable, and not optimizing the parameters perfectly
Neural networks or more precisely artificial neural networks	Works even if one or a few units fail to respond to the network	Referred to as "black box" models and provide very little insight, and require a large diversity of training datasets
Deep learning	Very accurate, can be adapted to many types of problems, and the hidden layers reduce the need for feature engineering	Requires a very large amount of data, and computationally intensive to train
Logistic regression	Have a nice probabilistic interpretation, and updated easily with new data	Not flexible enough to naturally capture more complex relationships
K-means	Fast, simple, and flexible	Manually specify the number of clusters
Ensembles (decision tree)	Perform very well, robust to outliers, and scalable	Unconstrained, and prone to overfitting
Principal component analysis	Versatile, fast, and simple to implement	Not interpretable, and manually set a threshold for a cumulative variance
Naive Bayes	Performs surprisingly well, easy to implement, and can scale with the dataset	Often beaten by models properly trained and tuned (algorithms listed)

Table 1.
Strengths and weaknesses of the most machine learning methods discussed here appearing in radiation oncology studies.

little insight) for large datasets [6, 13]. The development of accurate and interpretable models using different ML architectures is an active area of research [6]. As with any algorithm that we use in radiation oncology today (e.g., dose calculation or deformable registration), ML algorithms will need acceptance, commissioning, and QA to ensure that the right algorithm or model are applied to the right application and that the model results make sense in a given clinical situation. Finally, the field of radiation oncology is highly algorithmic and data-centric, and while the road ahead is filled with potholes, the destination holds tremendous promise [14].

3.3 How far are the reported results by the investigators correct?

The reported prediction results [15–38, 41–47, 52–60, 63–67, 71, 72, 74–77, 79–83, 85–88, 89–95, 97–102] by investigators indicate the performance of these predictive models on data that used in modeling. However, these ML models can suffer from different data biases which may lead to lack of generalizability. A machine learning system trained on local datasets only may not be able to predict (reproduce) the needs of out-of-sample datasets (new datasets that are not presented in the training data). External validation of models in cohorts, which were acquired independently from the discovery cohort (e.g., from another institution) is considered the gold standard for true estimates of performance and generalizability of prediction models [6]. The application of different algorithms to the same dataset may yield variable results for predictors found to be significantly associated with the outcome of interest [6, 105]. However, this may also suggest a potential limitation of self-critical assessment of published ML models or realistic confidence levels with implications for their practical clinical value [6].

3.4 How would the reported results be improved?

Although promising and improving accuracy results of many ML-based predictive models in radiation oncology have been reported [18, 19, 21, 31–38, 41–43, 53–55, 74, 79–83, 85, 86, 89–95, 97–102], the effective applications of these methods in day-to-day clinical practice are very few yet. Such an example of a recently deployed commercial product into clinical use is Quick Match (Siris Medical, Redwood City, CA, USA) [68]. A private initiative, such as IBM's Watson, is already used in some institutions such as the Memorial Sloan Kettering Cancer Center in New York [106–109]. Watson Oncology [108] is a cognitive AI computing system designed to support the broader oncology community of physicians as they consider treatment options with their patients. To improve the prediction accuracy of these reported results, more training and validation datasets from multi-institution are required. Such frameworks, e.g., [50] to compare these methods on standard consensus data to establish benchmarks for evaluating different models would definitely lead to improving these results and developing robust toolkits/systems. It is anticipated to see ML and AI tools very soon settled more effectively with the indispensable role in the routine clinical practice for the benefit of patients, society, and the profession.

3.5 Impact on automating the clinical process

The machine learning systems have been developed and deployed to do jobs on their own. Automated clinical processes in radiation oncology could be auto-piloted with driving technologies to execute automated tasks. For example, data-driven planning [63–67] is not fully automated at present as it requires expert oversight and/or intervention to ensure safely deliverable treatment plans. One challenge of achieving full automatic planning using reinforcement learning lies in the close integration and need for robust TPSs [14]. The future vision is toward a fully-automated planning process, from contouring to plan creation. Machine-based and patient-based virtual QA can have profound implications on the current IMRT/VMAT process. The automated process nature would definitely lead to expediting radiation oncology workflow and reduce the time burden of human intervention [62].

3.6 Impact on clinical decision-making support toward precision medicine in radiation oncology

ML tools for computer-aided detection/diagnosis [15–22] as "second opinion" systems for clinical decision-making support would undoubtedly enhance the radiologists' performance and hence improved diagnostic performance. The emerging paradigms in radiomics for therapeutic outcome predictions (i.e., patient's survival, decrease recurrence, late complication, etc.) [97–102] for individual patients would maximize its potential impact on precision radiotherapy. Individual patients can be stratified into subtypes based on radiomic biomarkers that contain information about cancer traits that determine the patient's prognosis [97]. Therefore, physicians may prescribe a more or less intense radiation regimen for an individual based on model predictions of local control benefit and toxicity risk [2], which would be considered for the optimal treatment planning design process and hence improving the quality of life for radiotherapy cancer patients. Effective implementation of adaptive radiation therapy with ML [85–88] can also further improve the precision in the radiotherapy treatments. The pre-planning prediction of dosimetric tradeoffs to assist physicians and patients to make better informed decisions about treatment modality and dose prescription [68] thus it can establish individualized and achievable goals. The clinical implications derived from personalized cancer therapy ensure not only that patients receive optimal treatment, but also that the right resources are being used for the right patients.

4. Conclusions

Machine learning methods used in radiation oncology workflow, from patient consult to follow-up, are presented and discussed in this chapter. Big data in radiation oncology, efforts made and current challenges, are addressed. With the era of big data, the utilization of machine learning algorithms in radiation oncology is growing fast. ML techniques could compensate for human limitations in handling a large amount of flowing information in an efficient manner, in which simple errors can make the difference between life and death. Machine learning is also indispensable in the radiomics scheme, characterization of image phenotypes of the tumor, with the potential for decision-making and precision medicine in radiation therapy by predicting treatment outcomes for individual patients rather than one-size-fits-all approach.

Acknowledgements

The author is grateful to the attending physicians, physicists, residents, and staff at the radiation oncology department, at American University of Beirut Medical Center (AUBMC), Lebanon. Most of the clinical aspects provided in this chapter were based on the author's knowledge and experience gained during his residency at AUBMC. The contents are solely representing the author's view. The author also specially thanks the IntechOpen for granting this chapter a full funding for Open-Access publication.

Conflict of interest

The author has no conflict of interest.

Author details

Alexander F.I. Osman
Department of Medical Physics, Al-Neelain University, Khartoum, Sudan

*Address all correspondence to: alexanderfadul@yahoo.com

References

[1] Halperin E, Brady L, Perez C, Wazer D. Perez and Brady's Principles and Practice of Radiation Oncology. 5th ed. Philadelphia: Lippincott Williams & Wilkins; 2008. 2106 p

[2] El Naqa I, Li R, Murphy M. Machine Learning in Radiation Oncology: Theory and Applications. Cham: Springer; 2015. 336 p. DOI: 10.1007/978-3-319-18305-3

[3] Kansagra AP, Yu JP, Chatterjee AR, Lenchik L, Chow DS, Prater AB, et al. Big data and the future of radiology informatics. Academic Radiology. 2016;**23**(1):30-42. DOI: 10.1016/j.acra.2015.10.004

[4] Lustberg T, van Soest J, Jochems A, Deist T, van Wijk Y, Walsh S, et al. Big data in radiation therapy: Challenges and opportunities. The British Journal of Radiology. 2017;**90**(1069):20160689. DOI: 10.1259/bjr.20160689

[5] Oberije C, Nalbantov G, Dekker A, Boersma L, Borger J, Reymen B, et al. A prospective study comparing the predictions of doctors versus models for treatment outcome of lung cancer patients: A step towards individualized care and shared decision making. Radiotherapy and Oncology. 2014;**112**:37-43. DOI: 10.1016/j.radonc.2014.04.012

[6] El Naqa I, Ruan D, Valdes G, Dekker A, McNutt T, Ge Y, et al. Machine learning and modeling: Data, validation, communication challenges. Medical Physics. 2018;**45**(10):e834-e840. DOI: 10.1002/mp.12811

[7] Mayo CS, Kessler ML, Eisbruch A, Weyburne G, Feng M, Hayman JA, et al. The big data effort in radiation oncology: Data mining or data farming? Advances in Radiation Oncology. 2016;**1**(4):260-271. DOI: 10.1016/j.adro.2016.10.001

[8] Chen RC, Gabriel PE, Kavanagh BD, McNutt TR. How will big data impact clinical decision making and precision medicine in radiation therapy? International Journal of Radiation Oncology, Biology, Physics. 2016;**95**(3):880-884. DOI: 10.1016/j.ijrobp.2015.10.052

[9] Benedict SH, Hoffman K, Martel MK, Abernethy AP, Asher AL, Capala J, et al. Overview of the American Society for Radiation Oncology-National Institutes of Health-American Association of Physicists in Medicine Workshop 2015: Exploring opportunities for radiation oncology in the era of big data. International Journal of Radiation Oncology, Biology, Physics. 2016;**95**:873-879. DOI: 10.1016/j.ijrobp.2016.03.006

[10] ACR Data Science InstituteTM to Guide Artificial Intelligence Use in Medical Imaging. 2017. Available at: https://www.acrdsi.org/-/media/DSI/Files/Strategic-Plan.pdf?la=en

[11] Alpaydin E. Introduction to Machine Learning. 3rd ed. Cambridge, MA: The MIT Press; 2014

[12] Ao S-I, Rieger BB, Amouzegar MA. Machine Learning and Systems Engineering. Dordrecht, NY: Springer; 2010

[13] Friedman J, Hastie T, Tibshirani R. The Elements of Statistical Learning. Vol. 1. Berlin: Springer; 2001

[14] Feng M, Valdes G, Dixit N, Solberg TD. Machine learning in radiation oncology: Opportunities, requirements, and needs. Frontiers in Oncology. 2018;**8**:110. DOI: 10.3389/fonc.2018.00110

[15] Suzuki K, Armato SG 3rd, Li F, Sone S, Doi K. Massive training artiicial neural network (MTANN) for reduction

of false positives in computerized detection of lung nodules in low-dose computed tomography. Medical Physics. 2003;**30**(7):1602-1617. DOI: 10.1118/1.1580485

[16] Chan HP, Lo SC, Sahiner B, Lam KL, Helvie MA. Computer-aided detection of mammographic micro-calcifications: Pattern recognition with an artificial neural network. Medical Physics. 1995;**22**(10):1555-1567. DOI: 10.1118/1.597428

[17] Zhu Y, Wang L, Liu M, Qian C, Yousuf A, Oto A, et al. MRI-based prostate cancer detection with high-level representation and hierarchical classification. Medical Physics. 2017;**44**(3):1028-1039. DOI: 10.1002/mp.12116

[18] Rezaei M, Yang H, Meinel C. Deep neural network with l2-norm unit for brain lesions detection. In: Liu D, Xie S, Li Y, Zhao D, El-Alfy ES, editors. Neural Information Processing. ICONIP 2017. Cham: Springer; 2017. pp. 798-807. DOI: 10.1007/978-3-319-70093-9_85

[19] Cheng JZ, Ni D, Chou YH, Qin J, Tiu CM, Chang YC, et al. Computer-aided diagnosis with deep learning architecture: Applications to breast lesions in US images and pulmonary nodules in CT scans. Scientific Reports. 2016;**6**:24454. DOI: 10.1038/srep24454

[20] Feng PH, Lin Y, Lo GM. A machine learning texture model for classifying lung cancer subtypes using preliminary bronchoscopic findings. Medical Physics. 2018;**45**(12):5509-5514. DOI: 10.1002/mp.13241

[21] Beig N, Khorrami M, Alilou M, et al. Perinodular and intranodular radiomic features on lung CT images distinguish adenocarcinomas from granulomas. Radiology. 2018;**290**(3):1-10. https://doi.org/10.1148/radiol.2018180910

[22] Joo S, Yang YS, Moon WK, Kim HC. Computer-aided diagnosis of solid breast nodules: Use of an artificial neural network based on multiple sonographic features. IEEE Transactions on Medical Imaging. 2004;**23**(10):1292-1300. DOI: 10.1109/TMI.2004.834617

[23] Valdes G, Luna JM, Eaton E, Simone CB II, Ungar LH, Solberg TD. MediBoost: A patient stratification tool for interpretable decision making in the era of precision medicine. Scientific Reports. 2016;**6**:37854. DOI: 10.1038/srep37854

[24] Caruana R, Lou Y, Gehrke J, Koch P, Sturm M, Elhadad N. Intelligible models for healthcare: Predicting pneumonia risk and hospital 30-day readmission. In: Proceedings of the 21th ACM SIGKDD International Conference on Knowledge Discovery and Data Mining. New York, USA: ACM; 2015. pp. 1721-1730. DOI: 10.1145/2783258.2788613

[25] Caruana R, Niculescu-Mizil A. An empirical comparison of supervised learning algorithms. In: Proceedings of the 23rd International Conference on Machine Learning. Pittsburgh: ACM; 2006. pp. 161-168. DOI: 10.1145/1143844.1143865

[26] Fernández-Delgado M, Cernadas E, Barro S, Amorin D. Do we need hundreds of classifiers to solve real world classification problems. Journal of Machine Learning Research. 2014;**15**:3133-3181

[27] Fayad H, Gilles M, Pan T, Visvikis D. A 4D global respiratory motion model of the thorax based on CT images: A proof of concept. Medical Physics. 2018;**45**(7):3043-3051. DOI: 10.1002/mp.12982

[28] Steiner E, Shieh C, Caillet V, O'Brien R, et al. WE-HI-KDBRB1-10: 4DCT and 4DCBCT under-predict intrafraction lung target motion during radiotherapy. Medical Physics. 2018;**45**(6):e646-e647. DOI: 10.1002/mp.12938

[29] Dick D, Wu X, Zhao W. MO-E115-GePD-F5-3: Fiducial-less tracking for the radiation therapy of liver tumors using artificial neural networks. Medical Physics. 2018;**45**(6):e415-e415. DOI: 10.1002/mp.12938

[30] Johansson A, Balter J, Cao Y. WE-AB-202-5: Gastrointestinal 4D MRI with respiratory motion correction. Medical Physics. 2018;**45**(6):e583-e583. DOI: 10.1002/mp.12938

[31] Nie D, Cao X, Gao Y, Wang L, Shen D. Estimating CT image from MRI data using 3D fully convolutional networks. In: Carneiro G et al., editors. Deep Learning and Data Labeling for Medical Applications. DLMIA 2016, LABELS 2016. LNCS. Vol. 10008. Cham: Springer; 2016. pp. 170-178. DOI: 10.1007/978-3-319-46976-8_18

[32] Bayisa F, Liu X, Garpebring A, Yu J. Statistical learning in computed tomography image estimation. Medical Physics. 2018;**45**(12):5450-5460. DOI: 10.1002/mp.13204

[33] Huynh T, Gao Y, Kang J, et al. Estimating CT image from MRI data using structured random forest and auto-context model. IEEE Transactions on Medical Imaging. 2016;**35**(1):174-183. DOI: 10.1109/TMI.2015.2461533

[34] Chen S, Qin A, Zhou D, Yan D. Technical note: U-net-generated synthetic CT images for magnetic resonance imaging-only prostate intensity-modulated radiation therapy treatment planning. Medical Physics. 2018;**45**(12):5659-5665. DOI: 10.1002/mp.13247

[35] Bahrami K, Shi F, Rekik I, Shen D. Convolutional neural network for reconstruction of 7T-like images from 3T MRI using appearance and anatomical features. In: Carneiro G et al., editors. Deep Learning and Data Labeling for Medical Applications. Cham, Switzerland: Springer, Verlag; 2016. pp. 39-47. DOI: 10.1007/978-3-319-46976-8_5

[36] Bahrami K, Shi F, Zong X, Shin HW, An H, Shen D. Reconstruction of 7T-like images from 3T MRI. IEEE Transactions on Medical Imaging. 2016;**35**(9):2085-2097. DOI: 10.1109/TMI.2016.2549918

[37] Bahrami K, Rekik I, Shi F, Gao Y, Shen D. 7T-guided learning framework for improving the segmentation of 3T MR images. Medical Image Computing and Computer-Assisted Intervention. 2016;**9901**:572-580. DOI: 10.1007/978-3-319-46723-8_66

[38] Bahrami K, Shi F, Rekik I, Gao Y, Shen D. 7T-guided super-resolution of 3T MRI. Medical Physics. 2017;**44**(5):1661-1677. DOI: 10.1002/mp.12132

[39] Guerrero T, Zhang G, Huang TC, Lin KP. Intrathoracic tumour motion estimation from CT imaging using the 3D optical flow method. Physics in Medicine and Biology. 2004;**49**(17):4147-4161

[40] Zhang T, Chi Y, Meldolesi E, Yan D. Automatic delineation of on-line head-and-neck computed tomography images: Toward on-line adaptive radiotherapy. International Journal of Radiation Oncology, Biology, Physics. 2007;**68**(2):522-530. DOI: 10.1016/j.ijrobp.2007.01.038

[41] Hu S, Wei L, Gao Y, Guo Y, Wu G, Shen D. Learning-based deformable image registration for infant MR images in the first year of life. Medical Physics. 2017;**44**(1):158-170. DOI: 10.1002/mp.12007

[42] Zagoruyko S, Komodakis N. Learning to compare image patches via convolutional neural networks. IEEE Conference on Computer Vision and Pattern Recognition. 2015:4353-4361. DOI: 10.1109/CVPR.2015.7299064

[43] Jiang D, Shi Y, Chen X, Wang M, Song Z. Fast and robust multimodal image registration using a local derivative pattern. Medical Physics. 2017;**44**(2):497-509. DOI: 10.1002/mp.12049

[44] Neylon J, Min Y, Low DA, Santhanam A. A neural network approach for fast, automated quantification of DIR performance. Medical Physics. 2017;**44**(8):4126-4138. DOI: 10.1002/mp.12321

[45] Wu J, Su Z, Li Z. A neural network-based 2D/3D image registration quality evaluator for pediatric patient setup in external beam radiotherapy. Journal of Applied Clinical Medical Physics. 2016;**17**(1):22-33. DOI: 10.1120/jacmp.v17i1.5235

[46] Wu G, Kim M, Wang Q, Munsell BC, Shen D. Scalable high-performance image registration framework by unsupervised deep feature representations learning. IEEE Transactions on Biomedical Engineering. 2016;**63**(7):1505-1516. DOI: 10.1109/TBME.2015.2496253

[47] Kearney V, Haaf S, Sudhyadhom A, Valdes G, Solberg TD. An unsupervised convolutional neural network-based algorithm for deformable image registration. Physics in Medicine and Biology. 2018;**63**(18):185017. DOI: 10.1088/1361-6560/aada66

[48] International Commisssion of Radiation Units and Measuremets. The ICRU Report 83: Prescribing, Recording and Reporting Photon-beam Intensity Modulated Radiation Therapy (IMRT). Oxford University Press; 2010. 107 p. DOI: 10.1093/jicru/ndq002

[49] Podgorsak EB. Radiation Oncology Physics: A Handbook for Teachers and Students. International Atomic Energy Agency (IAEA): IAEA; 2005. 657 p

[50] Menze BH, Jakab A, Bauer S, Kalpathy-Cramer J, Farahani K, et al. The multimodal brain tumor image segmentation benchmark (BRATS). IEEE Transactions on Medical Imaging. 2015;**34**(10):1993-2024. DOI: 10.1109/TMI.2014.2377694

[51] Bakas S, Akbari H, Sotiras A, Bilello M, Rozycki M, Kirby J, et al. Segmentation Labels and radiomic features for the pre-operative scans of the TCGA-GBM collection. The Cancer Imaging Archive. 2017. DOI: 10.7937/K9/TCIA.2017.KLXWJJ1Q

[52] Osman AFI. Automated brain tumor segmentation on magnetic resonance images and patient's overall survival prediction using support vector machines. In: Crimi A, Bakas S, Kuijf H, Menze B, Reyes M, editors. Brainlesion: Glioma, Multiple Sclerosis, Stroke and Traumatic Brain Injuries. Cham: Springer; 2018. pp. 435-449. DOI: 10.1007/978-3-319-75238-9_37

[53] Kamnitsas K, Bai W, Ferrante E, et al. Ensembles of multiple models and architectures for robust brain tumour segmentation. In: Crimi A, Bakas S, Kuijf H, Menze B, Reyes M, editors. Brain Les 2017. . LNCS. Vol. 10670. Cham: Springer; 2018. pp. 450-462. DOI: 10.1007/978-3-319-75238-9_38

[54] Kamnitsas K, Ledig C, Newcombe VF, et al. Efficient multi-scale 3D CNN with fully connected CRF for accurate brain lesion segmentation. Medical Image Analysis. 2017;**36**:61-78. DOI: 10.1016/j.media.2016.10.004

[55] Pereira S, Pinto A, Alves V, Silva CA. Brain tumor segmentation using convolutional neural networks in MRI images. IEEE Transactions on Medical Imaging. 2016;**35**(5):1240-1251. DOI: 10.1109/TMI.2016.2538465

[56] Guo Y, Gao Y, Shen D. Deformable MR prostate segmentation via deep feature learning and sparse patch matching. IEEE Transactions on Medical

Imaging. 2016;**35**(4):1077-1089. DOI: 10.1109/TMI.2015.2508280

[57] Men K, Dai J, Li Y. Automatic segmentation of the clinical target volume and organs at risk in the planning CT for rectal cancer using deep dilated convolutional neural networks. Medical Physics. 2017;**44**(12): 6377-6389. DOI: 10.1002/mp.12602

[58] Carass A, Roy S, Jog A, Cuzzocreo JL, Magrath E, Gherman A, et al. Longitudinal multiple sclerosis lesion segmentation: Resource and challenge. NeuroImage. 2017;**148**:77-102. DOI: 10.1016/j.neuroimage.2016.12.064

[59] Yang X, Wu N, Cheng G, Zhou Z, Yu DS, Beitler JJ, et al. Automated segmentation of the parotid gland based on atlas registration and machine learning: A longitudinal MRI study in head-and-neck radiation therapy. International Journal of Radiation Oncology, Biology, Physics. 2014;**90**(5):1225-1233. DOI: 10.1016/j.ijrobp.2014.08.350

[60] Ibragimov B, Xing L. Segmentation of organs-at-risks in head and neck CT images using convolutional neural networks. Medical Physics. 2017;**44**(2):547-557. DOI: 10.1002/mp.12045

[61] LeCun Y, Bengio Y, Hinton G. Deep learning. Nature. 2015;**521**(7553): 436-444. DOI: 10.1038/nature14539

[62] Thompson RF, Valdes G, Fuller CD, Carpenter CM, Morin O, Aneja S, et al. Artificial intelligence in radiation oncology: A specialty-wide disruptive transformation? Radiotherapy and Oncology. 2018;**129**(3):421-426. DOI: 10.1016/j.radonc.2018.05.030

[63] Nwankwo O, Mekdash H, Sihono DS, Wenz F, Glatting G. Knowledge-based radiation therapy (KBRT) treatment planning versus planning by experts: Validation of a KBRT algorithm for prostate cancer treatment planning. Radiation Oncology. 2015;**10**:111. DOI: 10.1186/s13014-015-0416-6

[64] Li N, Carmona R, Sirak I, Kasaova L, Followill D, Michalski J, et al. Highly efficient training, refinement, and validation of a knowledge-based planning quality-control system for radiation therapy clinical trials. International Journal of Radiation Oncology, Biology, Physics. 2017;**97**(1):164-172. DOI: 10.1016/j.ijrobp.2016.10.005

[65] Chatterjee A, Serban M, Abdulkarim B, Panet-Raymond V, Souhami L, Shenouda G, et al. Performance of knowledge-based radiation therapy planning for the glioblastoma disease site. International Journal of Radiation Oncology, Biology, Physics. 2017;**99**(4):1021-1028. DOI: 10.1016/j.ijrobp.2017.07.012

[66] Tol JP, Delaney AR, Dahele M, Slotman BJ, Verbakel WF. Evaluation of a knowledge-based planning solution for head and neck cancer. International Journal of Radiation Oncology, Biology, Physics. 2015;**91**(3):612-620. DOI: 10.1016/j.ijrobp.2014.11.014

[67] Foy JJ, Marsh R, Ten Haken RK, Younge KC, Schipper M, Sun Y, et al. An analysis of knowledge-based planning for stereotactic body radiation therapy of the spine. Practical Radiation Oncology. 2017;7(5):e355-e360. DOI: 10.1016/j.prro.2017.02.007

[68] Valdes G, Simone CB, Chen J, Lin A, Yom SS, et al. Clinical decision support of radiotherapy treatment planning: A data-driven machine learning strategy for patient-specific dosimetric decision making. Radiotherapy and Oncology. 2017;**125**(3):392-397. DOI: 10.1016/j.radonc.2017.10.014

[69] Zhu X, Ge Y, Li T, Thongphiew D, Yin FF, Wu Q J. A planning quality evaluation tool for prostate adaptive IMRT based on machine learning.

Medical Physics. 2011;**38**(2):719-726. DOI: 10.1118/1.3539749

[70] Moore KL, Schmidt R, Moiseenko V, Olsen LA, Tan J, Xiao Y, et al. Quantifying unnecessary normal tissue complication risks due to suboptimal planning: A secondary study of RTOG 0126. International Journal of Radiation Oncology, Biology, Physics. 2015;**92**(2):228-235. DOI: 10.1016/j.ijrobp.2015.01.046

[71] Rowbottom CG, Webb S, Oldham M. Beam-orientation customization using an artificial neural network. Physics in Medicine and Biology. 1999;**44**:2251. DOI: 10.1088/0031-9155/44/9/312

[72] Llacer J, Li S, Agazaryan N, Promberger C, Solberg TD. Non-coplanar automatic beam orientation selection in cranial IMRT: A practical methodology. Physics in Medicine and Biology. 2009;**54**(5):1337-1368. DOI: 10.1088/0031-9155/54/5/016

[73] Silver D, Huang A, Maddison CJ, Guez A, Sifre L, van den Driessche G, et al. Mastering the game of go with deep neural networks and tree search. Nature. 2016;**529**:484-489. DOI: 10.1038/nature16961

[74] Li Q, Chan MF. Predictive time-series modeling using artificial neural networks for Linac beam symmetry: An empirical study. Annals of the New York Academy of Sciences. 2017;**1387**(1): 84-94. DOI: 10.1111/nyas.13215

[75] El Naqa I. SU-E-J-69: An anomaly detector for radiotherapy quality assurance using machine learning. Medical Physics. 2011;**38**:3458. DOI: 10.1118/1.3611837

[76] Ford EC, Terezakis S, Souranis A, Harris K, Gay H, Mutic S. Quality control quantification (QCQ): A tool to measure the value of quality control checks in radiation oncology. International Journal of Radiation Oncology, Biology, Physics. 2012;**84**(3):e263-e269. DOI: 10.1016/j.ijrobp.2012.04.036

[77] Hoisak JD, Pawlicki T, Kim GY, Fletcher R, Moore KL. Improving linear accelerator service response with a real-time electronic event reporting system. Journal of Applied Clinical Medical Physics. 2014;**15**(5):4807. DOI: 10.1120/jacmp.v15i5.4807

[78] Huq MS, Fraass BA, Dunscombe PB, Gibbons JP Jr, Ibbott GS, et al. The report of task group 100 of the AAPM: Application of risk analysis methods to radiation therapy quality management. Medical Physics. 2016;**43**(7):4209. DOI: 10.1118/1.4947547

[79] Osman A, Maalej N, Jayesh K. SU-K-KDBRA1-01: A novel learning approach for predicting MLC positioning during dynamic IMRT delivery. Medical Physics. 2018;**45**(6):e357-e358. DOI: 10.1002/mp.12938

[80] Valdes G, Morin O, Valenciaga Y, Kirby N, Pouliot J, Chuang C. Use of TrueBeam developer mode for imaging QA. Journal of Applied Clinical Medical Physics. 2015;**16**(4):322-333. DOI: 10.1120/jacmp.v16i4.5363

[81] Valdes G, Scheuermann R, Hung CY, Olszanski A, Bellerive M, Solberg TD. A mathematical framework for virtual IMRT QA using machine learning. Medical Physics. 2016;**43**(7):4323. DOI: 10.1118/1.4953835

[82] Valdes G, Chan MF, Lim SB, Scheuermann R, Deasy JO, Solberg TD. IMRT QA using machine learning: A multi-institutional validation. Journal of Applied Clinical Medical Physics. 2017;**18**(5):279-284. DOI: 10.1002/acm2.12161

[83] Carlson JN, Park JM, Park SY, Park JI, Choi Y, Ye SJ. A machine learning

approach to the accurate prediction of multi-leaf collimator positional errors. Physics in Medicine and Biology. 2016;**61**(6):2514-2531. DOI: 10.1088/0031-9155/61/6/2514

[84] Liu C, Kim J, Kumarasiri A, Mayyasa E, Browna S, Wen N, et al. An automated dose tracking system for adaptive radiation therapy. Computer Methods and Programs in Biomedicine. 2018;**154**:1-8. DOI: 10.1016/j.cmpb.2017.11.001

[85] Guidi G, Maffei N, Meduri B, D'Angelo E, Mistretta GM, et al. A machine learning tool for re-planning and adaptive RT: A multicenter cohort investigation. Physica Medica. 2016;**32**(12):1659-1666. DOI: 10.1016/j.ejmp.2016.10.005

[86] Chetvertkov MA, Siddiqui F, Kim J, Chetty I, Kumarasiri A, Liu C, et al. Use of regularized principal component analysis to model anatomical changes during head and neck radiation therapy for treatment adaptation and response assessment. Medical Physics. 2016;**43**(10):5307-5319. DOI: 10.1118/1.4961746

[87] Tseng HH, Luo Y, Cui S, Chien JT, Ten Haken RK, Naqa IE. Deep reinforcement learning for automated radiation adaptation in lung cancer. Medical Physics. 2017;**44**:6690-6705. DOI: 10.1002/mp.12625

[88] Varfalvy N, Piron O, Cyr MF, Dagnault A, Archambault L. Classification of changes occurring in lung patient during radiotherapy using relative γ analysis and hidden Markov models. Medical Physics. 2017;**44**: 5043-5050. DOI: 10.1002/mp.12488

[89] Lee S, Ybarra N, Jeyaseelan K, Faria S, Kopek N, Brisebois P, et al. Bayesian network ensemble as a multivariate strategy to predict radiation pneumonitis risk. Medical Physics. 2015;**42**(5):2421-2430. DOI: 10.1118/1.4915284

[90] Naqa IE, Deasy JO, Mu Y, Huang E, Hope AJ, Lindsay PE, et al. Datamining approaches for modeling tumor control probability. Acta Oncologica. 2010;**49**(8):1363-1373. DOI: 10.3109/02841861003649224

[91] Zhen X, Chen J, Zhong Z, Hrycushko B, Zhou L, Jiang S, et al. Deep convolutional neural network with transfer learning for rectum toxicity prediction in cervical cancer radiotherapy: A feasibility study. Physics in Medicine and Biology. 2017;**62**(21):8246-8263. DOI: 10.1088/1361-6560/aa8d09

[92] Deist TM, Dankers FJWM, Valdes G, Wijsman R, Hsu IC, Oberije C, et al. Machine learning algorithms for outcome prediction in (chemo)radiotherapy: An empirical comparison of classifiers. Medical Physics. 2018;**45**(7):3449-3459. DOI: 10.1002/mp.12967

[93] Yahya N, Ebert MA, Bulsara M, House MJ, Kennedy A, Joseph DJ, et al. Statistical-learning strategies generate only modestly performing predictive models for urinary symptoms following external beam radiotherapy of the prostate: A comparison of conventional and machine-learning methods. Medical Physics. 2016;**43**(5):2040. DOI: 10.1118/1.4944738

[94] Zhang HH, D'Souza WD, Shi L, Meyer RR. Modeling plan-related clinical complications using machine learning tools in a multiplan IMRT framework. International Journal of Radiation Oncology, Biology, Physics. 2009;**74**(5):1617-1626. DOI: 10.1016/j.ijrobp.2009.02.065

[95] Kang J, Schwartz R, Flickinger J, Beriwal S. Machine learning approaches for predicting radiation therapy outcomes: A Clinician's perspective. International Journal of Radiation Oncology, Biology, Physics. 2015;**93**(5):1127-1135. DOI: 10.1016/j.ijrobp.2015.07.2286

[96] Baumann M, Krause M, Overgaard J, Debus J, Bentzen SM, Daartz J, et al. Radiation oncology in the era of precision medicine. Nature Reviews. Cancer. 2016;**16**(4):234-249. DOI: 10.1038/nrc.2016.18

[97] Arimura H, Soufi M, Kamezawa H, Ninomiya K, Yamada M. Radiomics with artificial intelligence for precision medicine in radiation therapy. Journal of Radiation Research. 2018;**60**(1):150-157. DOI: 10.1093/jrr/rry077

[98] Aerts HJ, Velazquez ER, Leijenaar RT, Parmar C, Grossmann P, et al. Decoding tumour phenotype by noninvasive imaging using a quantitative radiomics approach. Nature Communications. 2014;**5**:4006. DOI: 10.1038/ncomms5006

[99] Depeursinge A, Yanagawa M, Leung AN, Rubin DL. Predicting adenocarcinoma recurrence using computational texture models of nodule components in lung CT. Medical Physics. 2015;**42**(4):2054-2063. DOI: 10.1118/1.4916088

[100] Lambin P, Rios-Velazquez E, Leijenaar R, Carvalho S, van Stiphout RG, Granton P, et al. Radiomics: Extracting more information from medical images using advanced feature analysis. European Journal of Cancer. 2012;**48**(4):441-446. DOI: 10.1016/j.ejca.2011.11.036

[101] Wu J, Tha KK, Xing L, Li R. Radiomics and radiogenomics for precision radiotherapy. Journal of Radiation Research. 2018;**59**(suppl_1): i25-i31. DOI: 10.1093/jrr/rrx102

[102] Lao J, Chen Y, Li ZC, Li Q, Zhang J, Liu J, et al. A deep learning-based radiomics model for prediction of survival in glioblastoma multiforme. Scientific Reports. 2017;**7**:10353. DOI: 10.1038/s41598-017-10649-8

[103] Gulshan V, Peng L, Coram M, Stumpe MC, Wu D, Narayanaswamy A, et al. Development and validation of a deep learning algorithm for detection of diabetic retinopathy in retinal fundus photographs. The Journal of the American Medical Association. 2016;**316**:2402-2410. DOI: 10.1001/jama.2016.17216

[104] Mayo CS, Moran JM, Bosch W, Xiao Y, McNutt T, Popple R, et al. American Association of Physicists in Medicine Task Group 263: Standardizing nomenclatures in radiation oncology. International Journal of Radiation Oncology, Biology, Physics. 2018;**100**(4):1057-1066. DOI: 10.1016/j.ijrobp.2017.12.013

[105] Luo W, Phung D, Tran T, et al. Guidelines for developing and reporting machine learning predictive models in biomedical research: A multidisciplinary view. Journal of Medical Internet Research. 2016;**18**(12):e323. DOI: 10.2196/jmir.5870

[106] Parodi S, Riccardi G, Castagnino N, Tortolina L, Maffei M, Zoppoli G, et al. Systems medicine in oncology: Signaling network modeling and new generation decision-support systems. Methods in Molecular Biology. 2016;**1386**:181-219. DOI: 10.1007/978-1-4939-3283-2_10

[107] Memorial Sloan Kettering Cancer Center. Watson oncology. n.d. https://www.mskcc.org/about/innovative-collaborations/watson-oncology [Accessed: 30 January 2019]

[108] Kohn MS, Sun J, Knoop S, Shabo A, Carmeli B, Sow D, et al. IBM's health analytics and clinical decision support. Yearbook of Medical Informatics. 2014;**9**:154-162. DOI: 10.15265/IY-2014-0002

[109] Bibault JE, Giraud P, Burgun A. Big data and machine learning in radiation oncology: State of the art and future prospects. Cancer Letters. 2016;**382**(1):110-117. DOI: 10.1016/j.canlet.2016.05.033

Section 2

Image Processing in Medicine and Biology

Chapter 4

A Survey on 3D Ultrasound Reconstruction Techniques

Farhan Mohamed and Chan Vei Siang

Abstract

This book chapter aims to discuss the 3D ultrasound reconstruction and visualization. First, the various types of 3D ultrasound system are reviewed, such as mechanical, 2D array, position tracking-based freehand, and untracked-based freehand. Second, the 3D ultrasound reconstruction technique or pipeline used by the current existing system, which includes the data acquisition, data preprocessing, reconstruction method and 3D visualization, is discussed. The reconstruction method and 3D visualization will be emphasized. The reconstruction method includes the pixel-based method, volume-based method, and function-based method, accompanied with their benefits and drawbacks. In the 3D visualization, methods such as multiplanar reformatting, volume rendering, and surface rendering are presented. Lastly, its application in the medical field is reviewed as well.

Keywords: ultrasound, 3D reconstruction, position tracking technology, volume rendering, scientific visualization

1. Introduction

The medical imaging is very important for the physicians to visualize the inner anatomy of the patient for diagnosis and analysis purposes. There are various types of imaging modality, which are the magnetic resonance imaging (MRI), ultrasonography imaging, and computer tomography (CT) imaging. Recently, the use of ultrasound has become widely popular among the practitioners and researchers alike especially in the medical field, such as in obstetrics, in cardiology as well as in surgical guidance. This is due to the fact that the ultrasound is faster and safer, has noninvasive nature, and less expensive than the MRI and CT.

The conventional way to use the ultrasound machine is that the physician moves the ultrasound probe over the subject's skin to examine the region of interest (ROI). The ultrasound probe will feed the input signal to the ultrasound machine to display the 2D ultrasound image on the screen output. The 2D ultrasound image shows the cross-sectional part of the ROI. By using the hand-eye coordination approach, the physician is able to form a mentally constructed volume of that ROI for examination of the organ features and also to estimate the volume of the ROI. However, the reliance of 2D ultrasound images during the ultrasound scanning session can present some of the limitations as follows [1]:

1. The decision-making in diagnosis and analysis is very time-consuming and can also lead to incorrect decision, as the physician needs to transform a set of 2D ultrasound frames to mentally create a 3D impression of ROI.

2. The organ volume measurement is less accurate and dependent on operator's skill because only simple measurement is used to calculate the dimension of a ROI.

3. Some ROIs, such as the viewing of planes that are parallel to the skin, are difficult to visualize. This is due to the fact that movement of ultrasound probe is restricted when moving around the ROI.

On the other hand, 3D ultrasound volume can enhance the understanding of physicians to the scanned ROI without spending too much of mental workload. The 3D ultrasound volume visualization can be achieved by undergoing the 3D ultrasound reconstruction process, which is the generation of 3D ultrasound volume from a series of 2D ultrasound image. Before the 3D volume is reconstructed, data collection is required. There are several methods used for data acquisition, which are the 2D array scanning, mechanical scanning, tracked freehand scanning, and untracked freehand scanning. The data collected are generally comprised of the 2D ultrasound images and their relative spatial information.

After the data are obtained, the volume reconstruction method is implemented by using interpolation and approximation algorithm to get the 3D volume data and put them in a 3D volume grid based on the spatial information acquired from the tracking system. There are several methods of volume reconstruction method, such as pixel-nearest neighbor (PNN), voxel-nearest neighbor (VNN), distance weighted (DW), radial basis function (RBF), image-based algorithm, etc.

In order to visualize the reconstruction result, there are three basic types of rendering techniques, which are the surface rendering techniques, multiplanar reformatting techniques, and volume rendering techniques. This is the final stage for the 3D ultrasound reconstruction process where the physicians can view the 3D ultrasound data for analysis and diagnosis purposes, as well as for surgical guidance.

In terms of state-of-the-art approaches, many researchers also focused on the real-time 3D ultrasound imaging technology. In this way, the physicians are able to view the reconstruction results of the ROI immediately while scanning. Hence, the real-time 3D ultrasound can help the physicians to make decision efficiently and accurately as they can get an immediate feedback. Furthermore, the improvement in hardware devices, such as the graphical processing unit (GPU), also helps to achieve the goal of several research studies where the hardware limitation was an obstacle in the past.

This book chapter aims to present the current state of 3D ultrasound reconstruction and visualization techniques. The remainder of the book chapter is organized as follows. In Section 2, we will present the various 3D ultrasound imaging systems. In Section 3, the 3D ultrasound reconstruction process is described step by step. In Section 4, we present the application of 3D ultrasound in the medical application. We draw discussion and conclusion for future studies in Section 5. Although the ultrasound can be used in many other applications, such as in high-intensity focused ultrasound (HIFU) to kill cancer cell and to view crack in the wall and metal structure, etc., our scope is focused on the imaging or visualization of medical application.

2. 3D ultrasound imaging systems

The 3D ultrasound imaging system is a system that visualizes a ROI in 3D by reconstructing and combining a set of 2D ultrasound frames, which view from

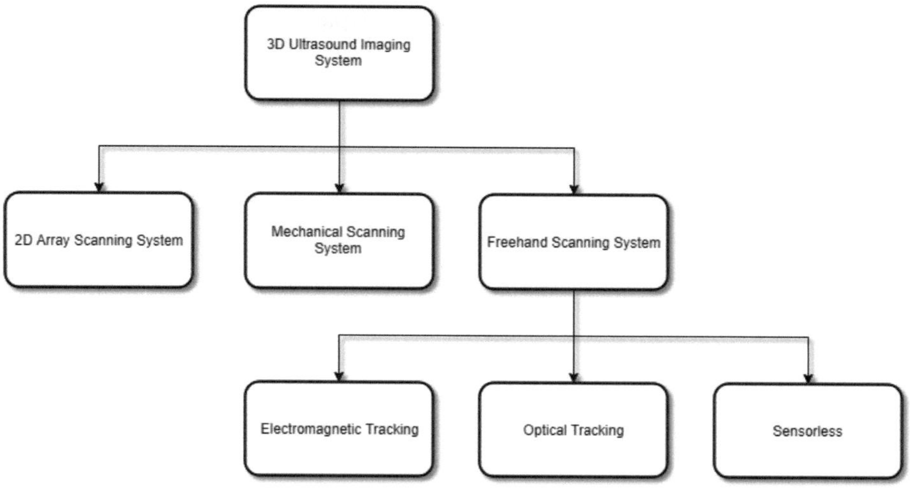

Figure 1.
The classification of 3D ultrasound imaging system.

different positions and angles of that ROI. The set of 2D ultrasound frames can be captured by different scanning methods or techniques as well as the transducer's dimensionality. **Figure 1** shows the classification of 3D ultrasound imaging system.

As data acquisition plays an important role in the accuracy and applicability of the 3D ultrasound volume reconstruction, selecting the most suitable 3D ultrasound imaging system is crucial. The choice is highly depended on the application, for example, the use of mechanical scanning system is suitable for transrectal ultrasound examination to evaluate the prostate gland in human body.

2.1 2D array transducer system

The 2D array scanning system used a dedicated 2D array ultrasound probe or 3D ultrasound probe that creates a pyramidal volume scan, which obtains a series of 2D ultrasound frames in real time [2]. Hence, it is able to create a time-dependent 3D ultrasound imaging system that can display the animation and flow visualization of the scanned ROI in between the scanning timeframe. It is the fastest way to view 3D ultrasound imaging in real time. As shown in **Figure 2**, the transducer elements are arranged in 2D array where each element fired an ultrasonic beam, which are combined to form a pyramidal volumetric scan. Hence, the transducer can remain stationery during ultrasound scanning session.

In contrast, 2D array scanning system is very expensive, is difficult to develop in terms of hardware and software, and is not commonly available [1, 4, 5]. Besides that, the transducer and ultrasound machine between different companies are not compatible to each other, due to the commercialized competition among the competitors [5]. Furthermore, the size of the acquired volume is limited by the geometric dimension of the transducer [3, 6].

2.2 Mechanical system

The 3D ultrasound image can also be obtained by the use of a cheaper linear array ultrasound probe, also known as the 2D ultrasound probe. This can be done by the transformation of a series of 2D ultrasound frames into a 3D ultrasound volume via the 3D ultrasound reconstruction process. These include the use of mechanical scanning system as well as freehand-based scanning system.

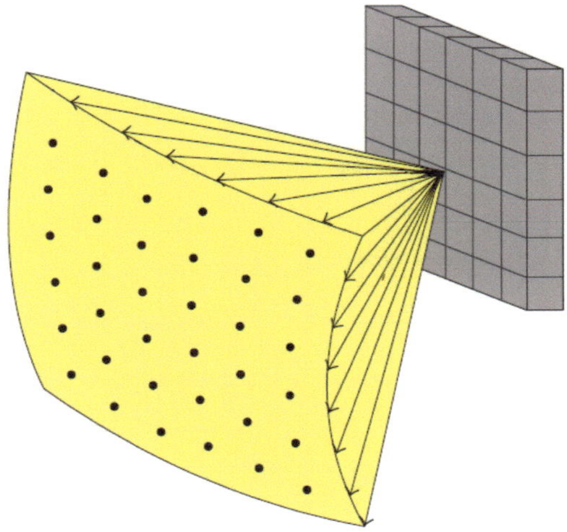

Figure 2.
The pyramidal volumetric scan of 2D array transducer [3].

The 3D mechanical probe consists of a linear array ultrasound probe, which is guided by a stepper motor inside a compact casing. The motor guides the ultrasound probe in a tilting, rotating, or linear movement around the ROI, as shown in **Figure 3**. When the motor is activated, multiple 2D ultrasound images can be acquired around the scanned ROI in a short time. Besides that, there is also a mechanical scanning system that uses a motorized mechanism and the external fixture, such as robot arm, to move the ultrasound probe. Both of the systems move the transducer in a predefined translation and orientation path around the ROI [4]. Therefore, this system is able to acquire regularly spaced 2D ultrasound frames [7] and also with accurate position and orientation that is relative to a frame [1]. These are the important factors to determine an accurate 3D ultrasound reconstruction image. However, mechanical scanning system is costly, not flexible, and angle of movement is limited because of its bulkiness size [3, 7].

2.3 Freehand-based system

The freehand-based scanning system acquires the 2D ultrasound images along with their position and orientation, by attaching a sensor on the ultrasound probe. The position tracking sensors are such as the electromagnetic sensor and the optical sensor. This system allows the operator to use the probe to scan around the desired ROI arbitrarily and hence is more flexible in terms of mobility than aforementioned

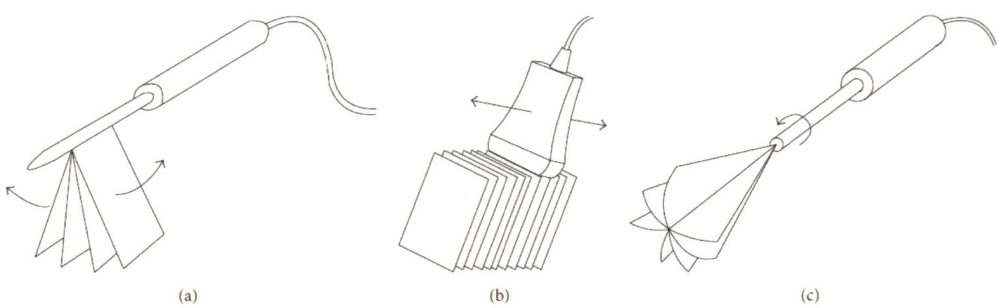

Figure 3.
Schematic diagram of 3D mechanical ultrasound probe scanning methods [3]: (a) tilting scanning; (b) linear scanning; (c) rotational scanning.

systems. Besides that, there exists a freehand-based scanning system that is without the use of position sensor. The advantages of freehand scanning system are low cost and scanning flexibility [4, 8]. On the downside, the 2D ultrasound frames acquired by freehand scanning system are usually irregular spacing between images and are highly sparse [9], which may cause undesired artifact in the reconstruction result. Therefore, the reconstruction methods or algorithms are researched and developed in order to solve the stated problem, which is further discussed in Section 3.3.

With the recent advancement of position tracking technology, the tracked freehand ultrasound scanning method has improved in terms of imaging quality, accuracy, effectiveness, portability, and reliability. Alternatively, the advancement of consumer-friendly hardware technologies introduced by the game industry not only can support better gaming experience but also provides a cost-effective solution to current problems, such as the use of Microsoft Kinect in healthcare sector [10]. The use of Sony's PlayStation (PS) Move and PS Eye are also proven to be useful in tracking positions in 3D space [11].

2.3.1 Electromagnetic-based position tracking

The electromagnetic tracking system is one of the popular types of freehand scanning system. Similar to the optical tracking system, this system also consists of two important components: the electromagnetic sensor mounted on the probe, as well as the electromagnetic transmitter, which tracks the position and orientation of that sensor on probe [4]. The recorded spatial information is then transferred to the computer workstation for reconstruction and visualization. However, electromagnetic tracking system suffers from the interference of magnetic signals if working nearby the sources, for example, surrounding metal instruments and power cables, which will affect the tracking accuracy [12], and also caused geometric distortion during the 3D reconstruction process [1].

2.3.2 Optical-based position tracking

The freehand 3D ultrasound imaging system with optical tracking sensor involves two important equipments: the markers mounted on the probe and one or multiple cameras to track the marker. Currently, the Polaris Optical Tracking System and Optotrak Certus are the two commercial optical trackers for 3D ultrasound imaging system and both are the product of Northern Digital (NDI). However, the problems found in the optical tracking system are that the marker mounted on the probe is large and caused the ultrasound scanning session to be inconvenient [12] and the line of sight of cameras must not be obstructed [13]. In order to counter this problem, the work in [13] created an optical tracking system with inertial sensor for freehand 3D ultrasound imaging, without external reference such as cameras. As for the cost-effective feature, in [11], the authors had introduced the use of PlayStation (PS) Move and PS Eye in the conventional 2D ultrasound probe for the 3D ultrasound reconstruction. This method is also able to offer portability and extensibility to the ultrasound imaging system.

2.3.3 Sensorless

The untracked freehand system or sensorless method requires the operator to move the transducer in a steady and regular motion at a constant linear or angular velocity, while 2D ultrasound frames are captured to generate a 3D ultrasound image [14]. Recently, a sensorless reconstruction method has been designed using a regression-based distance measurement, interpolation techniques, and unconstrained freehand data without any limitation on the trajectory [15]. In recent study, the image-based algorithm makes use of the adaptive speckle decorrelation to learn relative position and orientation between the acquired 2D ultrasound image pairs [16]. Since the sensorless freehand ultrasound does not need any position tracking sensor, it is considered the most portable 3D freehand ultrasound system [16]. However, the inconsistency scan rate and angle can cause the reconstruction result to be not smooth and also results in less quality 3D image during 3D visualization step [14].

3. 3D ultrasound reconstruction process

This section explained the 3D ultrasound reconstruction process in detail. This process is achieved from the use of 2D ultrasound probe with linear array. Based on [6], the standard workflow of the 3D ultrasound reconstruction is data acquisition stage, data preprocessing stage, volume reconstruction method stage, and 3D visualization stage. **Figure 4** shows the overall process of 3D ultrasound reconstruction.

3.1 Data acquisition

The data can be obtained from any ultrasound scanning systems that are presented in Section 2, such as sensorless system, electromagnetic tracking system, and optical tracking system. The obtained data are the 2D ultrasound frames and the orientation and position of the tracking sensor when a particular frame was taken. The B-scan image and its relative orientation and position must be synchronized [11]. As for the real-time system, there is a need to synchronize the image captured, position and orientation, and the time [17]. This synchronization process is also known as the temporal calibration [18].

Next, ultrasound probe calibration or spatial calibration is used to get the homogeneous transformation to convert each 2D coordinate pixel in 2D ultrasound frames into 3D coordinates voxel of ultrasound probe frame [12, 19, 20]. This method is used mostly in the real-time ultrasound 3D reconstruction system [19, 21].

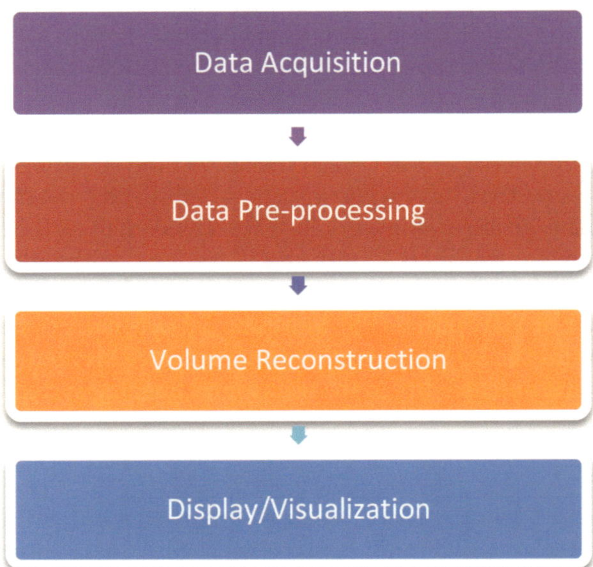

Figure 4.
The 3D ultrasound reconstruction process.

Scan conversion is also important for the reconstruction and visualization processes later, because of the possibility of different coordinate systems used by the scanning devices, such as in the work of [22], where the polar coordinate system recorded by the tracking system is converted into Cartesian coordinate system for 3D reconstruction. Besides that, reference [11] provides a method for the conversion of quaternion-based coordinate system into Cartesian coordinate system.

3.2 Data preprocessing

After the acquisition of the data, the data such as the 2D ultrasound frames are sent to the workstation for further processing. Most of the image processing techniques are used during this step, in order to enhance the 2D frames quality, remove noise, and preserve the edge boundary. This is because the 2D frames have various types of noise and artifacts, such as speckle noise, refraction, shadowing, reverberation, etc., and the spatial resolution within a 2D ultrasound frame is not uniform due to the transducer and signal characteristics varies with the penetration depth [7]. The example of image enhancement techniques included noise removing technique, histogram equalization, 2D Gaussian filter, median filtering, etc.

Figure 5 shows the noise and artifacts found in the 2D ultrasound frame. Besides that, segmentation process is also important to distinguish between the scanned objects in a region of interest (ROI), such as the skin, bone structure, etc., before the volume can be calculated. There are three types of segmentation process, which are automatic segmentation algorithms, semiautomatic segmentation algorithm, and manual segmentation. Automatic segmentation proves to be effective in obstetrics as the boundary of fetus and surrounding amniotic fluid is easy to be detected because of the high contrast between these two [6].

3.3 Volume reconstruction

The volume reconstruction methods are the most important part in the 3D ultrasound reconstruction process, which involved the implementation of interpolation and approximation algorithm to get the 3D volume data and put them in a 3D volume grid based on the spatial information acquired from the tracking system. The volume reconstruction also aims to reduce computational requirements without damaging or losing the underlying shape of the data [18]. Before the volume reconstruction methods start, the coordinate system and volume grid of reconstructed volume need to be established, such as volume size, axes of volume, origin of axes, and the size of voxel [23]. The volume coordinate configuration uses principal component analysis (PCA), which is a statistical tool that estimates the largest difference of collected data

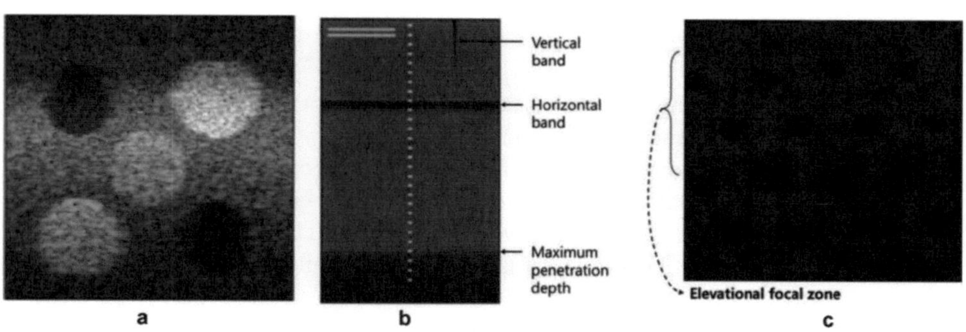

Figure 5.
Noise and artifacts [7]: (a) speckle noise; (b) transducer malfunction, and (c) elevational focal zone.

that the volume can enclose all the data values [23]. The bounding box technique is configured by computing the volume size by filling the voxel with pixels from a series of 2D ultrasound frames, and then the maximum point and the minimum point can be obtained. The bounding box is fast and simple to determine the volume coordinate configuration [8]. The minimum point is set as the origin of the volume. After the volume coordinate is configured, the volume reconstruction can be performed. There are several methods of volume reconstruction and they are pixel-based method (PBM), voxel-based method (VBM), and also function-based method (FBM). In addition, the Visualization Toolkit (VTK) is the most common software package for volume reconstruction and visualization, such as in [4, 11, 14, 16, 17, 24].

3.3.1 Pixel-based method (PBM)

The pixel-nearest neighbor (PNN) method is the example of pixel-based method (PBM), which is used to reconstruct the 3D volume by traveling across each pixel of acquired 2D ultrasound frames. In general, PNN consists of two important steps, which are bin-filling step and hole-filling step [25]. First, the bin-filling step is also known as distribution step and it travels across each pixel in all the 2D ultrasound frames, and then the nearest voxel in the 3D reconstructed volume is filled with that pixel value [4,8]. The method to assign pixel to voxel is based on the corresponding position and orientation information of 2D frames [9]. In this way, the 2D pixels can be transformed into voxels in the 3D volume space. If there have been multiple pixels assigned to a single voxel, the pixel values are averaged [4]. The bin-filling step might lead to empty voxel. Hence, hole-filing phase is used to identify and fill the empty voxel, usually by using the average, maximum, minimum, or a median of the neighbor filled voxels value [8, 9]. The selection of neighbor voxels is determined by a parameter value that represents the distance [24] or the radius of spherical region [8] from an empty voxel to be filled. However, the disadvantages of PNN method are causing blurred result and losing important information of 2D frames [9]. Besides that, some artifacts have been observed on the boundaries between the bin-filled area with original texture pattern and the hole-filled area with smoothed texture pattern [8].

Some research works are done in order to recover the disadvantages of PNN, especially in the hole-filling steps. Fast marching method (FMM) is proposed in the hole-filling step to interpolate empty voxel to preserve the sharp edges in the image and hence reduce the artifacts of the smoothed texture pattern [8]. Besides that, an improved Olympic operation is also proposed to estimate the empty voxel effectively [26]. Based on the observation, the PNN method is still favorable among the researchers in the field of 3D ultrasound reconstruction because of its simplicity to use as well as its capability to avoid complex computational time. Many improved PNN also has been proposed to create higher-quality reconstruction results.

3.3.2 Voxel-based method (VBM)

The voxel-based method (VBM) is used to reconstruct the 3D volume by traveling across each voxel in a volume grid and gathering the pixel values from input 2D ultrasound frames and computing them by various methods. The newly computed value is then placed at that voxel. The most common methods in VBM are voxel-nearest neighbor (VNN) and distance-weighted (DW). The VNN travels across each volume voxel and selects the nearest pixel value from a set of 2D frames to be put on that voxel. This method is capable to preserve the original texture patterns from 2D ultrasound frames; however, its downside is that large distance of the voxel to the 2D frames will generate large reconstruction artifacts and also it tends to preserve the speckle noise from corrupted ultrasound echo [8, 9].

As for the DW method, it also travels across each volume voxel first. Then, its local neighborhood pixels of 2D ultrasound frames are weighted by the inverse distances between the pixels and that voxel [27]. Lastly, the average value of those pixels is placed on the voxel. The DW method is able to suppress speckle noise [8]. On the other hand, it also smoothens the 3D reconstructed volume, causing the loss of some information on the original 2D ultrasound frames [9].

Besides that, the implementation of kernel regression can also help estimate the whole voxels in a volume, which is filled by bin-filling stage with more details and suppressing speckle noises, but it suffers from computational speed [9]. Although there is a use of bin-filling step, the use of kernel regression in this sense is considered a VBM as it also requires the reconstruction process to travel across each voxel in a volume.

3.3.3 Function-based method (FBM)

The functional-based method (FBM) takes a set of input data and uses a function like polynomial to reconstruct 3D ultrasound volume [28]. The radial basis function (RBF) is one of the FBMs that used an estimate function to compute a spline that passes through the pixels that form a shape in the 2D ultrasound frames [9, 27]. The created splines need to be as identical and smooth as the original shapes in the 2D frames. The approximation requirement is required because of the existence of measurement errors, as well as to reduce the overshoots in order to have the gray-level range of interpolated voxels to be same as that of the original 2D ultrasound frames [27]. The mentioned measurement errors are such as the tissue motion, position sensor error, and calibration error during the data acquisition process. In addition, the overshoot is a situation in signal processing where the signal or function exceeds its supposed target.

Besides RBF, Bayesian framework can be used to infer the voxel values in a volume grid by assuming a 3D parametric function that has basic function centered at every voxel, and the volume grid is modeled using piecewise smooth Markov random field (PS-MRF) with typical 6-connected neighborhood system [7, 29]. The work of [7] showed that the PS-MRF can work with irregular spaced B-scan images and to reduce the speckle noise and preserve boundary. However, it requires extreme computation time and needs to use GPU and parallel programming to overcome this limitation. The FBMs able to create a high-quality 3D volume from the 2D ultrasound frames; however, they require intensive computational power as well as speed, which imply that these methods are not widely studied in the field of 3D ultrasound reconstruction.

3.4 3D visualization

After volume reconstruction, the 3D visualization method is used to display the volume data from the volume gird for the operator and physicians to see the result of ultrasound scanning. This is useful for them to analyze the scanned anatomy and assist in diagnosis, as well as for image-guided surgery. The 3D visualization process is also the last step to complete the fully functioning 3D ultrasound reconstruction. The common rendering algorithms or techniques for 3D visualization are multiplanar reformatting, volume rendering, and surface rendering.

3.4.1 Multiplanar reformatting

The multiplanar reformatting method is a visualization technique where 2D ultrasound planes, also known as resliced image, are extracted from the 3D ultrasound

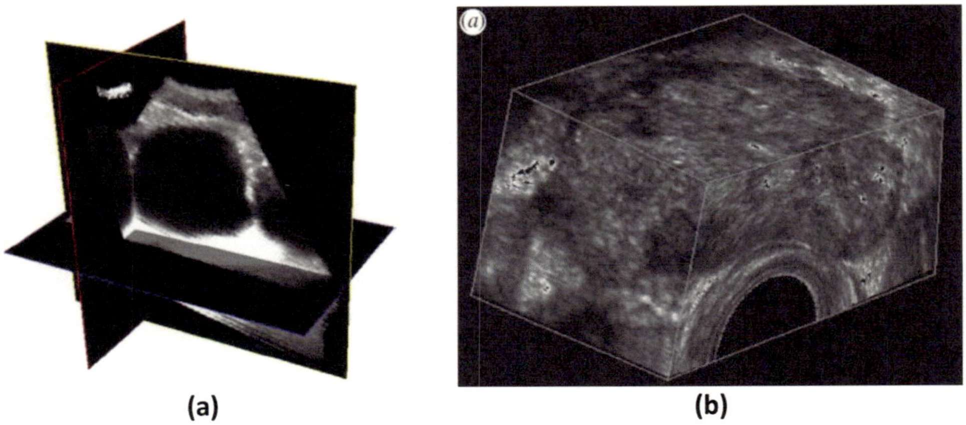

Figure 6.
(a) Planar cross-sectional images of reconstructed volume data [8] and (b) cube view of reconstructed volume data [1].

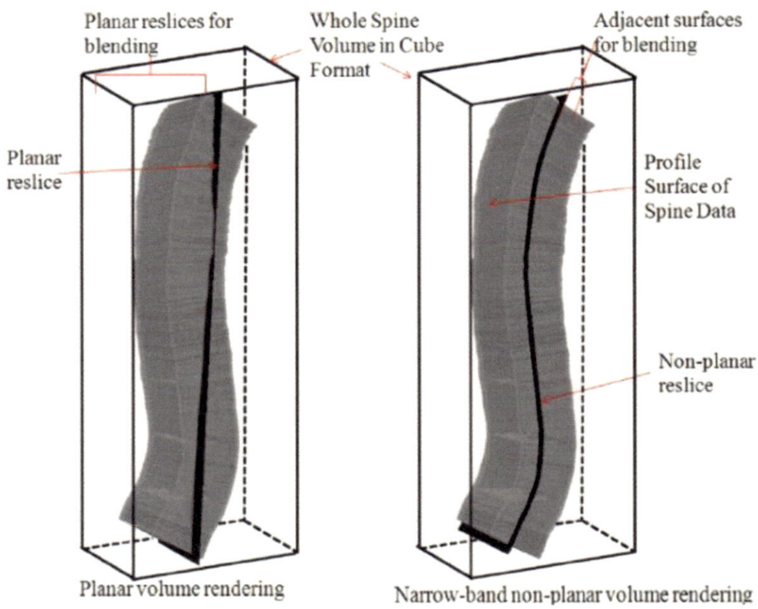

Figure 7.
The example shows the difference of planar and nonplanar volume rendering in the assessment of scoliosis [31].

data and displayed to the user with 3D impression [30]. The physicians can view the 3D ultrasound reconstruction result on three orthogonal slice views, which is in terms of traverse plane, coronal plane, and sagittal plane [17]. The resliced images are presented together with texture-mapped 3D rendering. There are three approaches of display [1], which are the planar cross-sectional images, the cube view, and the orthogonal planes. The limitation of planar viewing is that there will be possibility to loss of information due to the complex shape of ROI, especially when viewing spinal curvature. Thus, the use of nonplanar volume rendering method can compensate this limitation [31]. Due to its simplicity and the fact that it does not require high computational power, the multiplanar reformatting method is favorable among researchers and practitioners alike to visualize the 3D ultrasound reconstruction. **Figure 6** shows the examples of planar cross-sectional images and the cube view, while **Figure 7** shows the difference between planar and nonplanar volume rendering.

3.4.2 Volume rendering

Volume rendering technique involves ray-casting or ray-marching techniques where the change of light that went through the 3D volume data is projected as the output visualization results for the operator to view [32]. The light absorption principle [33] is implemented in the volume rendering technique where every voxel has the attributes such as brightness, transparency, and color [30]. So, there are several approaches used for the volume rendering visualization, and they are maximum intensity projection and translucency rendering [1]. The volume rendering can distinguish between tissue and fluids very well, and hence, it is suitable to view 3D ultrasound fetal image [1, 32]. However, the volume rendering is CPU-intensive and is not suitable to view the soft tissues details [1]. **Figure 8** shows the ray-casting in volume rendering technique, and **Figure 9** shows the example of volume rendering that uses maximum and minimum intensity projection.

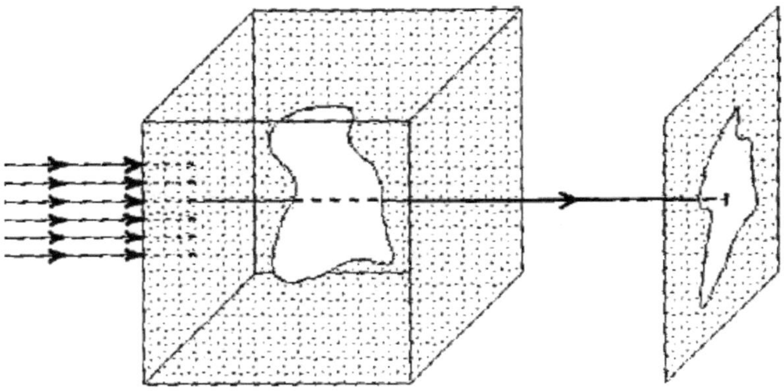

Figure 8.
The volume rendering technique involves several rays passing through 3D volume data. The synthesis methods can be applied to each voxel value that the ray passed to produce specific effects, such as transparency and maximum intensity projection of certain objects [32], such as tissues, blood vessels, etc.

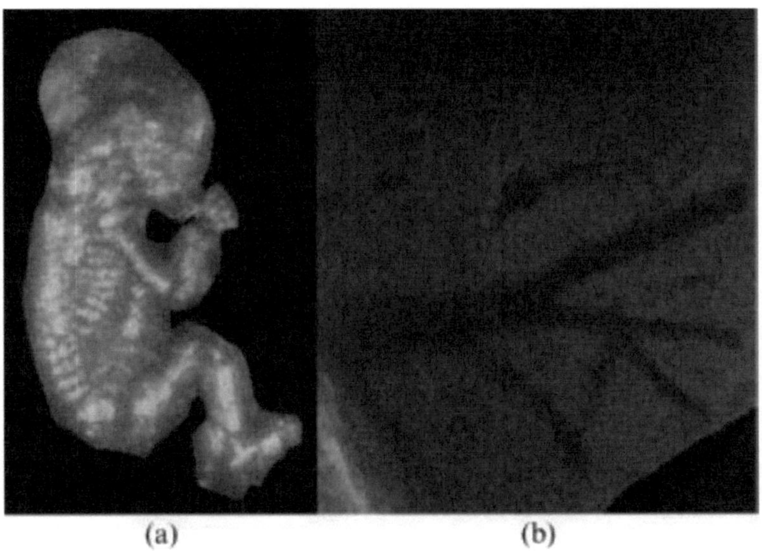

Figure 9.
The different volumes rendering visualization of 3D ultrasound imaging system approaches, where (a) shows the maximum intensity projection of a fetus and (b) shows the minimum intensity projection of blood vessels in the liver [30].

3.4.3 Surface rendering

The surface rendering produces a 3D surface based on the segmented boundary data points by generating the surface triangles or polygons associated with standard surface-rendering techniques being provided by interpolation [34]. The surface rendering can improve the interpretation of data sets [14]. The surface rendering technique can be classified into indirect surface rendering and direct surface rendering. The direct surface rendering is a special case of volume rendering technique, where the surface is rendered directly from the volume without intermediate geometric representations, setting thresholds or using object labels to define a range of voxel intensities to be viewed [35]. The transparency and colors are used for the better 3D visualization of the volume [36]. As for the indirect surface rendering, it requires that the surfaces of relevant structure boundaries within the volume be identified a priori by segmentation [35]. The example of indirect surface rendering is such as contour filtering and marching cubes. **Figure 10** shows the 3D visualization using surface rendering technique.

Contour filtering decides how contours of two successive slices to be connected where the vertices of the assigned contours should be connected to form triangular mesh [37]. This method is first introduced by Keppel [37] that used the triangulation for 3D surface rendering of contour lines from the medical data slices. The method is then optimized in the work of [38] using simplification algorithm to improve the level of detail as well as rendering speed.

Marching cubes algorithm is also one of the popular surface reconstruction algorithms introduced by Lorensen and Cline to display high-quality surface rendering for medical 3D volume data. The marching cubes algorithm uses a divide-and-conquer method [39] in a 3D volume data where the 3D volume is divided into many voxel cubes that form a voxel array. Each cube is made from eight vertices, which represents a voxel value from the volume data. A user-specific parameter value known as isovalue is defined before reconstruction in order to create a surface, also known as isosurface, by determining how the surface intersects with the cube [39]. Therefore, the surface rendering of different parts of the medical data, such as the arteries and atrium of the heart, can be distinguished and visualized,

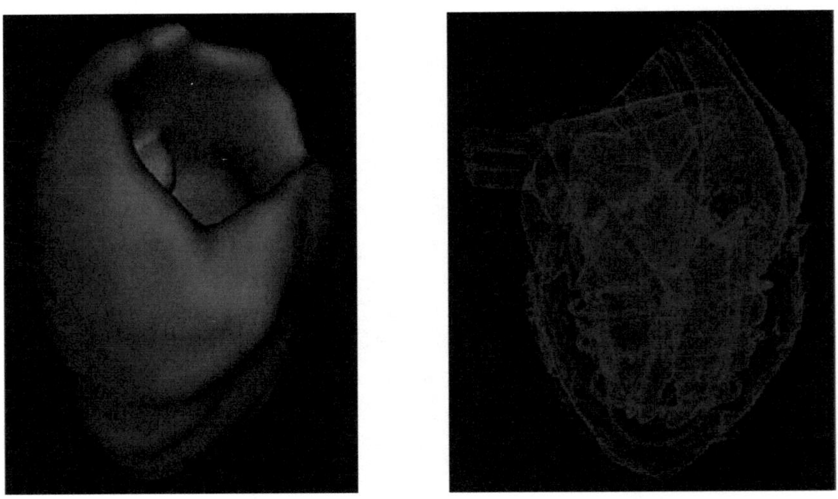

(a) (b)

Figure 10.
(a) The indirect surface rendering of cardiac structure [35] and (b) the direct surface rendering of an MR heart phantom [35].

as shown in **Figure 10(b)**. Then, the marching cubes process is moved to the next cube by following the order from left to right, front to back, and top to bottom until the algorithm ends [24]. In the marching cubes algorithm process, each vertex is assigned to a binary number either 1 or 0, where 1 means that the vertex is outside the surface, while 0 means that the vertex is inside the surface. In general, there are 2^8 = 256 cases on how surface intersects in a voxel cube, since eight vertices are

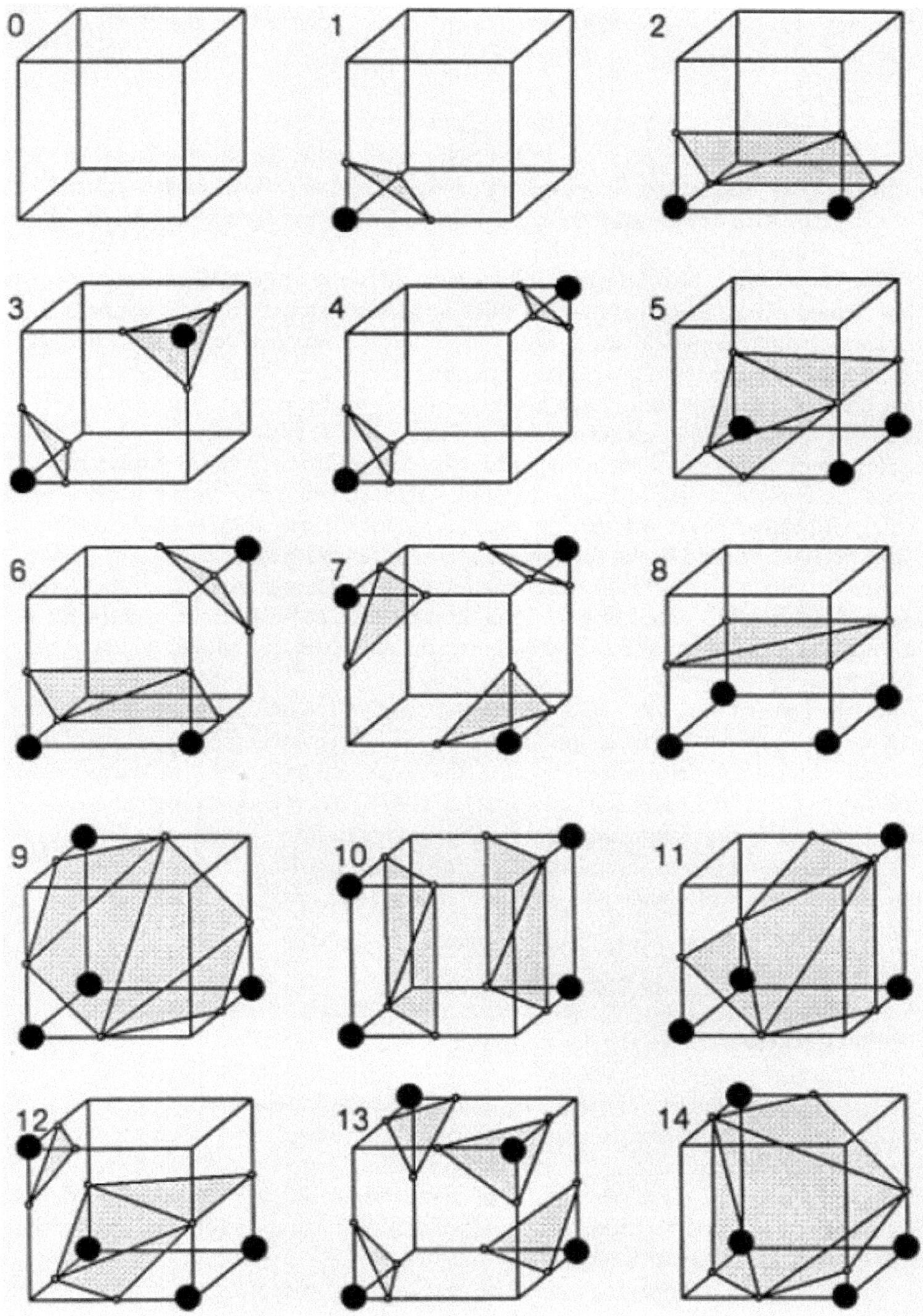

Figure 11.
The 15 unique pattern configurations [39].

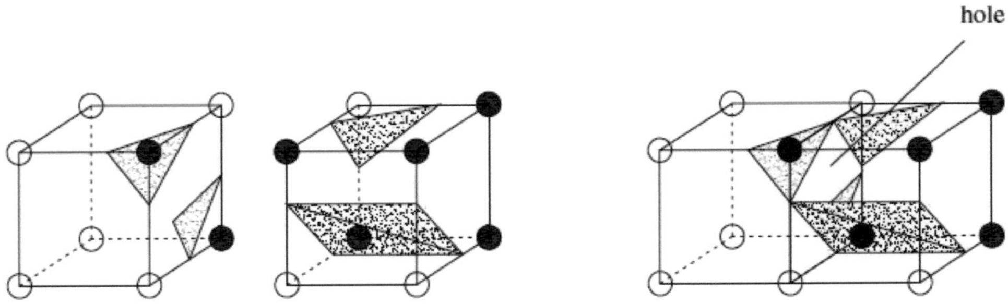

Figure 12.
The "hole problem" [40].

contained in a cube and are represented as binary number. Due to the fact that some of the cases are the inverse or symmetry of each other, the 256 cases are reduced into 15 cases with unique pattern configuration [33] and are put in a lookup table. The 15 unique pattern configurations are as shown in **Figure 11**.

The marching cubes algorithm has been implemented in the 3D reconstruction of medical data, such as in medical imaging reconstruction and creating a 3D contour of a mathematical scalar field [40] and in CT reconstruction [24]. Because of the utilization of lookup table, the marching cubes algorithm is fast and simple to use. It is also capable to take full advantage of the graphical processing unit (GPU) acceleration function to create good 3D reconstruction result [24].

However, the original marching cubes algorithm suffers from the connectivity problems between triangle of adjacent cubes also known as the "hole problem" [40], which will cause the reconstruction result to be not smooth. **Figure 12** shows the "hole problem" found in the conventional marching cubes algorithm. In order to solve this issue, the efforts have been made by the past researchers, such as modifying the lookup table, extending the look-up table, etc. In [40] introduced the 21 unique pattern configurations that will always ensure the triangles of adjacent cubes will connect to each other.

By the comparison, Wan et al. [14] found out that the marching cubes algorithm can produce sharper 3D ultrasound reconstruction image when compared with the contour filtering algorithm. Besides that, the result using marching cubes algorithm is easier to detect the edges and inner part of the ROI. However, the conventional marching cubes algorithm can generate a very large number of triangles for the 3D visualization [38]. In summary, marching cubes algorithm trades off speed for higher level of detail, while contour filtering sacrifices some details for computational speed.

4. Application of 3D ultrasound reconstruction in the medical visualization

The improvement of data acquisition methods, 3D reconstruction algorithms, volume visualizations, and hardware capabilities has greatly increased the feasibility of 3D ultrasound imaging in clinical application. Hence, the 3D ultrasound imaging has become more relevant in the medical field due to the increase in flexibility, efficiency, and real time applicability. In this section, the clinical application of 3D ultrasound reconstruction is discussed.

The 3D ultrasound imaging used in obstetrics brings two main advantages. Firstly, 3D ultrasound imaging can be used to determine the number of fetuses, fetus' surface feature, and placenta location [41]. The volume rendering can distinguish between tissue and surrounding amniotic fluids very well, and hence it is suitable to view 3D

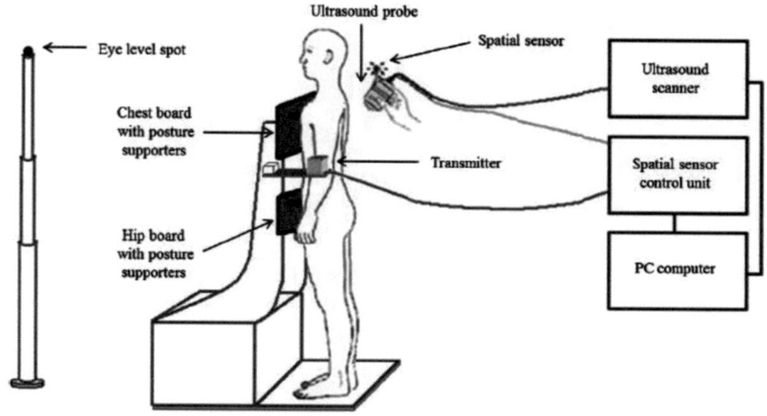

Figure 13.
The schematic diagram for the assessment of scoliosis using 3D ultrasound imaging system [31].

ultrasound fetal image for the physicians to examine the fetal presentation, as well as for the parents to see the fetus' face [1, 32]. It also can reduce the repeatability of physicians to relocate the placenta location and reduce mental workload to mentally construct the 2D ultrasound images into volumetric view. The second advantage is 3D ultrasound imaging that can assist in the accurate volume measurement of fetal size. Based on the World Health Organization (WHO) [41], the physicians need to measure the femur length, abdominal circumference, biparietal diameter, and head circumference, in order to determine whether the fetal is oversized or undersized.

In cardiology, 3D ultrasound imaging can help to identify the plague in blood vessel, such as atherosclerotic stenosis. This can be achieved using segmentation method to get the surface of the blood vessel [12].

Besides that, the 3D ultrasound imaging also proved to be effective in the assessment of scoliosis [31, 42]. Due to the need to follow up treatment frequently during the early stage, frequent X-ray examination is harmful for the young patient. Hence, 3D ultrasound reconstruction can help in scoliosis examination as ultrasound has less radiation generation and nontraumatic to the subject. The flexibility of ultrasound also allows the subject to be scanned in standing posture, which is more accurate to measure the spinal curvature angle as shown in **Figure 13**.

5. Conclusions

This chapter discussed the analysis on the literature of existing 3D ultrasound reconstruction method or algorithm. First, the 3D ultrasound imaging system can be classified as the 2D array scanning system, the mechanical scanning system, and the freehand scanning system. Their properties, advantages, and disadvantages are discussed. Second, the reconstruction process for the 3D ultrasound imaging system is explained. The steps required by the 3D ultrasound reconstruction are data acquisition stage, data preprocessing stage, implementing volume reconstruction method stage, and 3D visualization stage. Lastly, the advantages of 3D ultrasound reconstruction in the medical visualization are discussed, which includes obstetrics, cardiology, and scoliosis assessment.

The main limitation found in the current methods is the requirement for large computational processing power in order to visualize accurate medical data. Through the improvement of hardware capabilities such as GPU, the computational power and speed limitation can be improved. However, this presents a new problem, which is the increase in the cost of production. Therefore, we observed that the computational speed, accuracy of reconstruction, and cost-effectiveness are the challenges to be faced to provide a practicable 3D ultrasound reconstruction system.

In the future, the augmented reality (AR) medical can solve a lot of issue in ultrasonography, especially in the viewing of ultrasound image, as it can display the ultrasound image or other important information in the field of view of the physicians. This can further improve the clinician's perception toward the scanned ROI.

Furthermore, the data visualization method can also greatly improve the ultrasound perception by assigning the color to the scanned organs. This is because the current ultrasound images are black and white and are very hard to distinguish between different organs. Based on the physical properties of organs, the reflected intensity of ultrasonic wave is different for every organ. In this way, the color mapping can be used in different intensities to produce colorful ultrasound image, which represents and distinguishes every organ in the scanned region. Besides that, flow visualization can also be incorporated in the ultrasound visualization, such as different colors for different blood flow directions.

Acknowledgements

This chapter is supported by Ministry of Science, Technology & Innovation under the ScienceFund grant vote R.J130000.7928.4S135. The authors also like to acknowledge University of Technology, Malaysia (UTM) for providing the guidance to the research facilities to work.

Conflict of interest

This book chapter does not have any conflict of interest.

Author details

Farhan Mohamed and Chan Vei Siang*
Faculty of Engineering, School of Computing, University of Technology Malaysia (UTM), Johor Bahru, Johor, Malaysia

*Address all correspondence to: vschan2@live.utm.my

References

[1] Fenster A, Parraga G, Bax J. Three-dimensional ultrasound scanning. Interface Focus. 2011;**1**(June):503-519

[2] Fenster A, Downey DB, Cardinal HN. Three-dimensional ultrasound imaging. Physics in Medicine and Biology. 2001;**46**(5):R67. Available from: http://stacks.iop.org/0031-9155/46/i=5/a=201

[3] Huang Q, Zeng Z. A review on real-time 3D ultrasound imaging technology. BioMed Research International. 2017;**2017**:6027029. Available from: https://www.ncbi.nlm.nih.gov/pubmed/28459067

[4] Daoud MI, Alshalalfah A-L, Awwad F, Al-Najar M. Freehand 3D ultrasound imaging system using electromagnetic tracking. In: 2015 International Conference on Open Source Software Computing. 2015. pp. 1-5

[5] Jiang T, Yin L. 3D/4D cardiac ultrasound image registration from low cost 2D ultrasound instrument. Proceedings of 2012 IEEE-EMBS International Conference on Biomedical and Health Informatics, vol. 25. 2012. pp. 354-356

[6] Gee A, Prager R, Treece G, Berman L. Engineering a freehand 3D ultrasound system. Pattern Recognition Letters. 2003;**24**(4-5):757-777

[7] Moon H, Ju G, Park S, Shin H. 3D freehand ultrasound reconstruction using a piecewise smooth Markov random field. Computer Vision and Image Understanding. 2016;**151**:101-113. Available from: http://dx.doi.org/10.1016/j.cviu.2015.12.009

[8] Wen T, Zhu Q, Qin W, Li L, Yang F, Xie Y, et al. An accurate and effective FMM-based approach for freehand 3D ultrasound reconstruction. Biomedical Signal Processing and Control. 2013;**8**(6):645-656

[9] Chen X, Wen T, Li X, Qin W, Lan D, Pan W, et al. Reconstruction of freehand 3D ultrasound based on kernel regression. Biomedical Engineering Online. 2014;**13**(1):124. Available from: http://biomedical-engineering-online.biomedcentral.com/articles/10.1186/1475-925X-13-124

[10] Kitsunezaki N, Adachi E, Masuda T, Mizusawa JI. KINECT applications for the physical rehabilitation. In: MeMeA 2013—IEEE International Symposium on Medical Measurements and Applications, Proceedings. 2013. pp. 294-299

[11] Mohamed F, Mong WS, Yusoff YA. Quaternion based freehand 3D baby phantom reconstruction using 2D ultrasound probe and game controller motion and positioning sensors. In: International Conference for Innovation in Biomedical Engineering and Life Sciences, vol. 56. 2015. pp. 272-278

[12] Chung S-W, Shih C-C, Huang C-C. Freehand three-dimensional ultrasound imaging of carotid artery using motion tracking technology. Ultrasonics. 2017;**74**:11-20. Available from: http://linkinghub.elsevier.com/retrieve/pii/S0041624X16302001

[13] Goldsmith AM, Pedersen PC, Szabo TL. An inertial-optical tracking system for portable, quantitative, 3D ultrasound. In: Proceedings of the IEEE Ultrasonics Symposium. 2008. pp. 45-49

[14] Wan MH, Tan K, Supriyanto E. Development of 3D image reconstruction based on untracked 2D fetal phantom ultrasound images using VTK. WSEAS Transactions on Signal Processing. 2010;**6**(4):145-154. Available from: http://www.wseas.us/e-library/transactions/signal/2010/88-127.pdf

[15] Housden RJ, Gee AH, Treece GM, Prager RW. Sensorless reconstruction of freehand 3D ultrasound data. Medical Image Computing and Computer-Assisted Intervention. 2006;**9**(Pt 2):356-363

[16] Gao H, Huang Q, Xu X, Li X. Wireless and sensorless 3D ultrasound imaging. Neurocomputing. 2016;**195**:159-171. Available from: http://dx.doi.org/10.1016/j.neucom.2015.08.109

[17] Gobbi DG, Peters TM. Interactive intra-operative 3D ultrasound reconstruction and visualization. Medical Image Computing and Computer-Assisted Intervention. 2002;**2489**(2489):156-163. Available from: http://www.springerlink.com/content/nglmpkbb52lgjcl4

[18] Mozaffari MH, Lee W-S. Freehand 3-D ultrasound imaging: A systematic review. Ultrasound in Medicine & Biology. 2017;**43**(10):2099-2124. Available from: http://linkinghub.elsevier.com/retrieve/pii/S0301562917302776

[19] Chen TK, Thurston AD, Moghari MH, Ellis RE, Abolmaesumi P. A real-time ultrasound calibration system with automatic accuracy control and incorporation of ultrasound section thickness. SPIE. 2008;**2**:69182A-1-69182A-11. Available from: http://proceedings.spiedigitallibrary.org/proceeding.aspx?articleid=1329768

[20] Prager RW, Rohling RN, Gee AH, Berman L. Rapid calibration for 3-D freehand ultrasound. Ultrasound in Medicine & Biology. 1998;**24**(6):855-869

[21] Prager RW, Gee A, Berman L. Stradx: Real-time acquisition and visualization of freehand three-dimensional ultrasound. Medical Image Analysis. 1999;**3**(2):129-140

[22] Abdellak M, Abdelaziz A, Eldeib A. Interactive high resolution reconstruction of 3D ultrasound volumes on the GPU. In: Proceedings of the International Symposium on Biomedical Imaging; 2016–June. 2016. pp. 494-497

[23] San José-Estépar R, Martín-Fernández M, Caballero-Martínez PP, Alberola-López C, Ruiz-Alzola J. A theoretical framework to three-dimensional ultrasound reconstruction from irregularly sampled data. Ultrasound in Medicine & Biology. 2003;**29**(2):255-269

[24] Wang H, Pu X. 3D medical CT images reconstruction based on VTK and visual C++. In: 3rd International Conference on Bioinformatics and Biomedical Engineering (iCBBE 2009). 2009. pp. 1-4

[25] Dewi DEO, Wilkinson MHF, Mengko TLR, Purnama IKE, Van Ooijen PMA, Veldhuizen AG, et al. 3D ultrasound reconstruction of spinal images using an improved olympic hole-filling method. In: International Conference on Instrumentation, Communication, Information Technology, and Biomedical Engineering 2009, ICICI-BME 2009. New York: IEEE (The Institute of Electrical and Electronics Engineers); 2009. pp. 350-354

[26] Dewi DEO, TLR M, Purnama IKE, Veldhuizen AG, MHF W. An improved Olympic hole-filling method for ultrasound volume reconstruction of human spine. International Journal of E-Health and Medical Communications. 2010;**1**(3):28-40

[27] Rohling R, Gee A, Berman L. A comparison of freehand three-dimensional ultrasound reconstruction techniques. Medical Image Analysis. 1999;**3**(4):339-359

[28] Lindseth F, Langø T, Selbekk T, Hansen R, Reinertsen I, Askeland C, et al. Ultrasound-based guidance and therapy. Advancements and Breakthroughs in Ultrasound Imaging. 2013;(June):28-82. Available from: http://www.intechopen.com/books/advancements-and-breakthroughs-in-ultrasound-imaging/ultrasound-based-guidance-and-therapy

[29] Sanches JM, Marques JS. A Rayleigh reconstruction/interpolation algorithm for 3D ultrasound. Pattern Recognition Letters. 2000;**21**(10):917-926. Available from: http://www.sciencedirect.com/science/article/pii/S0167865500000532

[30] Prager RW, Ijaz UZ, Gee AH, Treece GM. Three-dimensional ultrasound imaging. Proceedings of the Institution of Mechanical Engineers. Part H, Journal of Engineering in Medicine. 2010;**224**(2):193-223. Available from: http://journals.sagepub.com/doi/10.1243/09544119JEIM586

[31] Cheung CJ, Zhou G, Law S, Mak T. Ultrasound volume projection imaging for assessment of scoliosis. IEEE Transactions on Medical Imaging. 2015;**34**(8):1760-1768

[32] Downey DB, Fenster A, Williams JC. Clinical utility of three-dimensional US. Radiographics. 2000;**20**(2):559-571. Available from: http://pubs.rsna.org/doi/10.1148/radiographics.20.2.g00mc19559

[33] Tan J, Chen J, Wang Y, Li L, Bao Y. Design of 3D visualization system based on vtk utilizing marching cubes and ray casting algorithm. In: Proceedings of the 8th International Conference on Intelligent Human-Machine Systems and Cybernetics (IHMSC) 2016; vol. 2. 2016. pp. 192-197

[34] Barry CD, Allott CP, John NW, Mellor PM, Arundel PA, Thomson DS, et al. Three-dimensional freehand ultrasound: Image reconstruction and volume analysis. Ultrasound in Medicine & Biology. 1997;**23**(8):1209-1224

[35] Zhang Q, Eagleson R, Peters TM. Volume visualization: A technical overview with a focus on medical applications. Journal of Digital Imaging. 2011;**24**(4):640-664

[36] Parmar BN, Bhatt T. Volume visualization using marching cubes algorithms: Survey & analysis. International Journal of Innovative Research in Technnology. 2016;**2**(11):21-25

[37] Keppel E. Approximating complex surfaces by triangulation of contour lines. IBM Journal of Research and Development. 1975;**19**(1):2-11. Available from: http://ieeexplore.ieee.org/articleDetails.jsp?arnumber=5391253

[38] Klein R, Schilling A, Straßer W. Reconstruction and simplification of surfaces from contours. Graph Models. 2000;**62**(6):429-443

[39] Lorensen WE, Cline HE. Marching cubes: A high resolution 3D surface construction algorithm. Computer Graphics (ACM). 1987;**21**(4):163-169

[40] Masala GL, Golosio B, Oliva P. An improved marching cube algorithm for 3D data segmentation. Computer Physics Communications. 2013;**184**(3):777-782. Available from: http://dx.doi.org/10.1016/j.cpc.2012.09.030

[41] World Health Organization (WHO). WHO Recommendations on Antenatal Care for a Positive Pregnancy Experience: Summary [Internet]. Geneva, Switzerland: World Health Organization; 2018. Available from: http://apps.who.int/iris/bitstream/

handle/10665/259946/WHO-RHR-18.01-eng.pdf; http://apps.who.int/iris/bitstream/10665/259946/1/WHO-RHR-18.01-eng.pdf

[42] Nguyen DV, Vo QN, Le LH, Lou EHM. Validation of 3D surface reconstruction of vertebrae and spinal column using 3D ultrasound data—A pilot study. Medical Engineering and Physics. 2015;**37**(2):239-244. Available from: http://linkinghub.elsevier.com/retrieve/pii/S1350453314002951

Section 3

Emerging Paradigms of Machine Learning

Chapter 5

Quantum Neural Machine Learning: Theory and Experiments

Carlos Pedro dos Santos Gonçalves

Abstract

Cloud-based access to quantum computers opens up the way for the empirical implementation of quantum artificial neural networks and for the future integration of quantum computation in different devices, using the cloud to access a quantum computer. The current work experimentally implements quantum artificial neural networks on IBM's quantum computers, accessed via cloud. Examples are provided for the XOR Boolean function representation problem and decision under risk; in the last case, quantum object-oriented programming using IBM's Qiskit Python library is employed to implement a form of quantum neural reinforcement learning applied to a classical decision under risk problem, showing how decision can be integrated into a quantum artificial intelligence system, where an artificial agent learns how to select an optimal action when facing a classical gamble. A final reflection is provided on quantum robotics and a future where robotic systems are connected to quantum computers via cloud, using quantum neural computation to learn to optimize tasks and act accordingly.

Keywords: quantum artificial neural networks, quantum neural reinforcement learning, quantum object-oriented programming, decision under risk

1. Introduction

Research on quantum neural machine learning has, until recently, mostly been a theoretical effort, anticipating a future where quantum computers would become available and sufficiently advanced to support quantum neural machine learning [1–5]. However, we now have quantum computers that are capable of implementing quantum artificial neural networks (QUANNs) experimentally, and one is able to access these computers via cloud. This brings QUANNs from the purely theoretical realm to the experimental realm, setting up the new stage for the expansion of quantum connectionism. In the current chapter, we address this issue, by implementing different QUANNs on IBM's quantum computers using the IBM Q Experience cloud-based access.

The chapter is divided into three sections. In Section 2, we address the basic properties of quantum neural computation, the connection with the quantum circuit computation model, and how different interpretations of quantum mechanics may address the basic computational dynamics involved.

In Section 3, we discuss how the IBM quantum computers can be considered QUANNs, illustrating with an example of a QUANN applied to the problem of the XOR Boolean function computation, implemented experimentally on two of IBM's devices (Section 3.1); afterward (Section 3.2), we turn to the experimental implementation of quantum robotics and quantum decision with a more complex form of quantum neural computation in the form of a variant of quantum neural reinforcement learning (QNRL), applied to a problem of decision under risk, where the agent must learn the optimal action that leads to the highest expected reward in a classical gamble.

The problem is first addressed in terms of the fundamental equations which employ quantum adaptive computation, namely quantum adaptive gates; then, we implement it experimentally on IBM's quantum computers and, afterward, we address the main Python code that was used to run the algorithm on these computers, thus, introducing quantum object-oriented programming (QOOP) and reflecting on its relevance for research on quantum artificial intelligence.

While, in Section 3.1, the main goal is to illustrate the implementation of QUANNs in a case where QUANNs exhibit a greater efficiency over classical ANNs, in Section 3.2, our main goal is not to address the speed-up of quantum algorithms over classical ones or even the greater efficiency of quantum algorithms over classical ones, but rather to provide for a reflection on the first steps for a possible future where quantum computation is incorporated in different (classical) robotic systems by way of the internet of things and cloud-based access to quantum devices, and the role that quantum adaptive computation may play in such a future.

In particular, in Section 3.2, we illustrate how a QUANN can become adaptive with respect to a problem that is given to it, in this case, a decision problem under risk, therefore, allowing us to address how QOOP can be employed to simulate an artificial agent, with a QUANN as its cognitive architecture, that must make a decision when presented a problem of classical decision under risk; therefore, our main goal in Section 3.2, from a computer science standpoint, is to address how a quantum artificially intelligent system decides when faced with a classical decision under risk problem, using QUANNs and QOOP.

In Section 4, we conclude with a chapter review and a reflection on future directions for cloud-based quantum-enabled technologies and QOOP.

2. Quantum neural computation and quantum mechanics

In order to address quantum neural computation, we need to first introduce some notation, which is commonly used in quantum computation, namely, we use the standard Dirac's *bra-ket* notation, where a *ket* vector corresponds to a column vector and the *bra* vector is its conjugate transpose. Defining, then, the fundamental *ket* vectors $|0\rangle$ and $|1\rangle$, respectively, as:

$$|0\rangle = \begin{pmatrix} 1 \\ 0 \end{pmatrix}, |1\rangle = \begin{pmatrix} 0 \\ 1 \end{pmatrix} \tag{1}$$

with the corresponding *bra* vectors $\langle 0|$ and $\langle 1|$ being defined, respectively, as the conjugate transpose of $|0\rangle$ and $|1\rangle$, then, we can represent Pauli's operators as:

$$\hat{\sigma}_1 = |0\rangle\langle 1| + |1\rangle\langle 0| = \begin{pmatrix} 0 & 1 \\ 1 & 0 \end{pmatrix} \tag{2}$$

$$\hat{\sigma}_2 = -i|0\rangle\langle 1| + i|1\rangle\langle 0| = \begin{pmatrix} 0 & -i \\ i & 0 \end{pmatrix} \tag{3}$$

$$\hat{\sigma}_3 = |0\rangle\langle 0| - |1\rangle\langle 1| = \begin{pmatrix} 1 & 0 \\ 0 & -1 \end{pmatrix} \tag{4}$$

The unit operator on the two-dimensional Hilbert space, spanned by the basis $\{|0\rangle, |1\rangle\}$, is denoted by $\hat{1} = |0\rangle\langle 0| + |1\rangle\langle 1|$ which has the form of the identity matrix.

The Walsh-Hadamard transform unitary operator is, in turn, given by:

$$\hat{U}_{WH} = \frac{\hat{\sigma}_1 + \hat{\sigma}_3}{\sqrt{2}} = \frac{1}{\sqrt{2}}\begin{pmatrix} 1 & 1 \\ 1 & -1 \end{pmatrix} \tag{5}$$

We also use the usual notation for the ket vectors $|+\rangle = \hat{U}_{WH}|0\rangle$ and $|-\rangle = \hat{U}_{WH}|1\rangle$.

Besides the above notation, we denote the binary alphabet by $A_2 = \{0, 1\}$ and the set of d-length binary strings by A_2^d, using boldface letters to represent binary strings of length greater than 1.

Using this notation, we are now ready to address some basic general properties of quantum neural computation.

The basic computational unit of a QUANN is a neuron with a two-level firing dynamics that can be described by the neural firing operator [5, 6]:

$$\hat{\nu} = \frac{\hat{1} - \hat{\sigma}_3}{2}\nu \tag{6}$$

where ν is a neural firing frequency expressed in Hertz.

The eigenvectors for this operator are given by:

$$\hat{\nu}|s\rangle = s\nu|s\rangle, s = 0, 1 \tag{7}$$

Therefore, the eigenvector $|0\rangle$ corresponds to a neural activity where the firing frequency is 0 Hz, while the eigenvector $|1\rangle$ corresponds to a neural activity where the firing frequency is 1 Hz. This means that there are two quantized energy levels associated with the artificial neuron, and these energy levels are obtained from the single neuron Hamiltonian, expressed in terms of the neural firing frequency operator as follows [5, 6]:

$$\hat{H} = 2\pi\eta\hat{\nu} \tag{8}$$

Therefore, the eigenvector $|0\rangle$ is associated with a neural firing energy level of 0 Joules, while the eigenvector $|1\rangle$ is associated with a neural firing energy level of $2\pi\eta\nu$ Joules.

For a neural network with d neurons, the neural firing activity can be addressed in terms of a neural field in the network, with the firing frequency field operators such that the k-th neuron neural firing operator $\hat{\nu}_k$ obeys the eigenvalue equation:

$$\hat{\nu}_k|s_1 s_2 ... s_d\rangle = s_k\nu|s_1 s_2 ... s_d\rangle \tag{9}$$

and any pair of neural firing operators commute; that is, for $k, l = 1, 2, ..., d$, $[\hat{\nu}_k, \hat{\nu}_l] = 0$. Thus, the total neural firing frequency operator is given by:

$$\hat{\nu}_{Tot} = \sum_{k=1}^{d} \hat{\nu}_k \tag{10}$$

which leads to the eigenvalue spectrum for the neural network:

$$\hat{\nu}_{Tot}|s_1 s_2 ... s_d\rangle = \sum_{k=1}^{d} s_k\nu|s_1 s_2 ... s_d\rangle \tag{11}$$

The general computational dynamics of a d-neuron QUANN can be addressed, in the quantum circuit model, by a computational chain of unitary operators, where the networked computation is implemented by conditional unitary operators that follow the structure of the neural links [4–6], which means that not all conditional unitary operators can be implemented in the neural network, but only those that respect the network's topology and processing direction.

Formally, then, an N-length computational chain that propagates forward in a quantum neural computation circuit is comprised of a sequential product of unitary operators:

$$\hat{C} = \hat{U}_N \hat{U}_{N-1} ... \hat{U}_1 \tag{12}$$

The sequence is read from right to left and such that $\hat{U}_1$ is the first operator to be applied and $\hat{U}_N$ is the last. This is the forward sequence proceeding from the beginning to the end of the computation. The reverse chain, which propagates backward in the computational circuit, is, then, given by the conjugate transpose of the forward chain:

$$\hat{C}^\dagger = \hat{U}_1^\dagger ... \hat{U}_{N-1}^\dagger \hat{U}_N^\dagger \tag{13}$$

Formally, given a general initial density operator, representing the initial neural field dynamics of the QUANN, expressed as follows:

$$\hat{\rho}_{in} = \sum_{\mathbf{r},\, \mathbf{s} \in \mathrm{A}_2^d} \rho_{\mathbf{r},\mathbf{s}} |\mathbf{r}\rangle\langle\mathbf{s}| \tag{14}$$

the quantum computation can be addressed in terms of the propagation:

$$\begin{aligned} \hat{\rho}_{out} &= \hat{C}\hat{\rho}\hat{C}^\dagger = \\ &= \sum_{\mathbf{r}',\, \mathbf{s}' \in \mathrm{A}_2^d} \left(\sum_{\mathbf{r},\, \mathbf{s} \in \mathrm{A}_2^d} \rho_{\mathbf{r},\mathbf{s}} \left\langle \mathbf{r}' \middle| \hat{U}_N \hat{U}_{N-1} ... \hat{U}_1 \middle| \mathbf{r} \right\rangle |\mathbf{r}'\rangle \left\langle \mathbf{s}' \right| \left\langle \mathbf{s} \middle| \hat{U}_1^\dagger ... \hat{U}_{N-1}^\dagger \hat{U}_N^\dagger \middle| \mathbf{s}' \right\rangle \right) \end{aligned} \tag{15}$$

The firing patterns, in Eq. (15), $\mathbf{r}$ and $\mathbf{s}$ correspond to input neural firing patterns for the QUANN, while the firing patterns $\mathbf{r}'$ and $\mathbf{s}'$ correspond to output neural firing patterns; in this way, the quantum neural computation is propagating in both directions of the computational chain, so that we have the propagation from the input to the output (from the beginning to the end of the computational chain), which corresponds to the amplitude $\langle \mathbf{r}' | \hat{U}_N \hat{U}_{N-1} ... \hat{U}_1 | \mathbf{r} \rangle$, and the propagation from the output to the input (from the end to the beginning of the computational chain), which corresponds to the amplitude $\left\langle \mathbf{s} \middle| \hat{U}_1^\dagger ... \hat{U}_{N-1}^\dagger \hat{U}_N^\dagger \middle| \mathbf{s}' \right\rangle$.

For the cases where there is a mismatch between the final output firing dynamics, that is, when $\mathbf{r}' \neq \mathbf{s}'$, the QUANN does not reach a well-defined output; from a computational perspective, we can state that the network does not reach a final solution, since the output computed in the forward direction of the computational circuit, $\langle \mathbf{r}' | \hat{U}_N \hat{U}_{N-1} ... \hat{U}_1 | \mathbf{r} \rangle$, does not match the output computed in the reverse direction of the computational circuit, $\left\langle \mathbf{s} \middle| \hat{U}_1^\dagger ... \hat{U}_{N-1}^\dagger \hat{U}_N^\dagger \middle| \mathbf{s}' \right\rangle$.

However, when $\mathbf{r}' = \mathbf{s}'$, the output computed in the forward and backward directions matches; this leads to the diagonal components of the final density operator that, for each $\mathbf{s}' \in \mathrm{A}_2^d$, are given by:

$$\left\langle \mathbf{s}' | \hat{\rho}_{out} | \mathbf{s}' \right\rangle | \mathbf{s}' \rangle \langle \mathbf{s}' | = \left(\sum_{\mathbf{r}, \mathbf{s} \in A_2^d} \rho_{\mathbf{r}, \mathbf{s}} \left\langle \mathbf{s}' | \hat{U}_N \hat{U}_{N-1} \ldots \hat{U}_1 | \mathbf{r} \right\rangle \left\langle \mathbf{s} \middle| \hat{U}_1^\dagger \ldots \hat{U}_{N-1}^\dagger \hat{U}_N^\dagger \middle| \mathbf{s}' \right\rangle \right) | \mathbf{s}' \rangle \langle \mathbf{s}' | \tag{16}$$

This means that the neural field computes each alternative final firing pattern $\mathbf{s}' \in A_2^d$ with a projective intensity given by the weighted sum over each pair of alternative initial firing patterns propagated in both directions of the computational chain:

$$\left\langle \mathbf{s}' | \hat{\rho}_{out} | \mathbf{s}' \right\rangle = \sum_{\mathbf{r}, \mathbf{s} \in A_2^d} \rho_{\mathbf{r}, \mathbf{s}} \left\langle \mathbf{s}' | \hat{U}_N \hat{U}_{N-1} \ldots \hat{U}_1 | \mathbf{r} \right\rangle \left\langle \mathbf{s} \middle| \hat{U}_1^\dagger \ldots \hat{U}_{N-1}^\dagger \hat{U}_N^\dagger \middle| \mathbf{s}' \right\rangle \tag{17}$$

From a computer science standpoint, this two-directional propagation, which is a basic result of the quantum circuit-based computation (generalizable to any type of quantum computer), exhibits a form of forward propagation and backward propagation, where the forward and backward amplitudes can be, from a computer science standpoint, addressed in terms of a probe and response dynamics, respectively; returning to Eq. (15), each amplitude $\langle \mathbf{r}' | \hat{U}_N \hat{U}_{N-1} \ldots \hat{U}_1 | \mathbf{r} \rangle$ can be addressed as a probing computational dynamics from the beginning to the end of the computational circuit that links the initial (input) firing pattern $\mathbf{r}$ to the final probed (output) firing pattern $\mathbf{r}'$, and the reverse amplitude $\left\langle \mathbf{s} \middle| \hat{U}_1^\dagger \ldots \hat{U}_{N-1}^\dagger \hat{U}_N^\dagger \middle| \mathbf{s}' \right\rangle$ can be addressed as a response that comes from the end of the computational circuit to the beginning, a response that links the output firing pattern $\mathbf{s}'$ to the initial input firing pattern $\mathbf{s}$.

When the two output firing patterns do not match, $\mathbf{r}' \neq \mathbf{s}'$, we have a mismatch between the probe and the response, and when the two firing patterns match, $\mathbf{r}' = \mathbf{s}'$, an *echo* is produced with an intensity given by the sum in Eq. (17); the computation is, then, like the search for the solution to a computational problem, where each probed alternative final output gets a response with a specific intensity.

These dynamics are simultaneous, that is, the QUANN processes in both the forward and backward directions simultaneously to arrive at the final result.

The above fundamental computational dynamics is characteristic of quantum mechanics, and not limited to QUANNs or quantum computation, nor is it dependent on one's interpretation of quantum mechanics. It arises when one considers the structure of a general density operator for a quantum system [6].

Indeed, as an example, let us consider a general density operator for a quantized observable $\hat{O}$ on some quantum system, which, for the purpose of illustration we consider to have a discrete, not necessarily finite, non-degenerate eigenvalue spectrum, so that the *ket* vectors $|m\rangle$, for $m = 0, 1, 2 \ldots$, satisfying $\hat{O}|m\rangle = o_m|m\rangle$, span the basis for a Hilbert space associated with the quantum system with respect to the observable; then, the general dynamics for the quantum system, with respect to the observable, can be represented as a density operator on the system's Hilbert space:

$$\hat{\rho} = \sum_{m, n} \rho_{m, n} |m\rangle \langle n| \tag{18}$$

The off-diagonal components of such an operator are such that there is no matching between the corresponding eigenvalues, only in the diagonal do we find a matching between the eigenvalues. The *ket* vector can, in this case, be considered as a probing vector, while the *bra* vector can be considered as a response vector.

In this way, only when a probed alternative eigenvalue finds a matching response eigenvalue do we have an *echo* for an alternative eigenvalue that can be actualized, and the probability for this actualization coincides with the diagonal density value $\rho_{m,m}$ which corresponds to the *echo intensity*. This is a basic result from quantum mechanics that extends to any observable, including observables with both discrete as well as continuous spectra.

It is important to stress that this *echo* dynamics is not specific to QUANNs, but is present in any quantum system; any density operator characterizing a quantum system exhibits, in the formalism, this main dynamics, so the *echo* dynamics is a characteristic of the physics of quantum systems and accounts for Born's probability rule in quantum mechanics—that is, the probability of an alternative eigenvalue to be observed is equal to the corresponding diagonal component of a density operator.

Therefore, embedded within quantum mechanics' formalism, we find an account of Born's probability rule. Furthermore, given a Hamiltonian operator for the quantum system $\hat{H}_S$, and a time lapse of Δt, quantum mechanics defines the unitary propagation of a density operator at time t_0 as:

$$\hat{\rho}(t_0 + \Delta t) = e^{-\frac{i}{\eta}\hat{H}_S\Delta t}\hat{\rho}(t_0)e^{\frac{i}{\eta}\hat{H}_S\Delta t} \tag{19}$$

In the case of the illustrative general example, given in Eq. (18), we get:

$$\hat{\rho}(t_0 + \Delta t) = \sum_{m,n}\left(\sum_{k,l}\rho_{k,l}(t_0)\langle m|e^{-\frac{i}{\eta}\hat{H}_S\Delta t}|k\rangle\langle l|e^{\frac{i}{\eta}\hat{H}_S\Delta t}|n\rangle\right)|m\rangle\langle n| \tag{20}$$

where $\langle m|\exp\left(-i/\eta\hat{H}_S\Delta t\right)|k\rangle$ is a forward in time propagating amplitude from the *k-th* initial eigenvalue to the *m-th* final eigenvalue and $\langle l|\exp\left(i/\eta\hat{H}_S\Delta t\right)|n\rangle$ is a backward in time propagating amplitude from the *n-th* final eigenvalue to the *l-th* initial eigenvalue[1], and this basic dynamics is a general result that stems from Schrödinger's unitary evolution.

Cramer was, however, the first to fully address the consequences of this dynamics and propose the concept of *echo*, within the context of quantum mechanics, addressing it related to Born's rule, deriving Born's rule from within the quantum formalism.

While Cramer [7] addresses the *echo* in terms of the encounter of a forward-propagating retarded wave (which we addressed above under the probe dynamics, proceeding forward from the beginning to the endpoint of the unitary evolution) and the backward-propagating advanced wave (which we addressed above under the response dynamics, proceeding from the endpoint to the beginning of the unitary evolution), by working with the density operator, instead of the wave function, we get a clearer picture of the corresponding dynamics, which accounts, in the case of any quantum physical system, for both the off-diagonal terms (as *failed echoes*) and the diagonal terms of the density operator (as the *echoes* where the probe was met by a matching response) with the *echo intensity* giving Born's probability rule. This result is generalizable and independent of the interpretation of quantum mechanics that one follows; that is, all interpretations of quantum mechanics agree with the above results.

It is important to clarify what an interpretation of quantum mechanics is and why there are different interpretations of the same theoretical body and equations. It turns out that the main interpretations do not disagree on the formalism,

---

[1] One may notice the change in the time lapse signal so that the conjugate transposition corresponds to time reversal.

methods, and how the mathematics is built and applied for prediction of experimental results. The interpretations do not stem from any ambiguity or lack of robustness in the formalism and in the application of the formalism, they stem from the fact that not everything is accounted for by the formalism, and that is where the interpretations come in.

To better frame this issue, one must consider the nature of the theory that one is dealing with, what it explains, and what is outside its theoretical scope.

Quantum mechanics is, in fact, a probabilistic theory of the quantized dynamics of fundamental physical fields, fields that work at the level of the building blocks of physical nature. The physical theory and methods that form the basic structure of quantum mechanics developed progressively from empirical observations and statistical findings on fundamentally random outcomes of physical experiments dealing with the quantum level.

This means that physicists found the basic rules for (dynamical) probability assignments that robustly capture the main probabilistic dynamics of quantum fields.

To understand the nature of the theory, it is important to stress that it was born out of laboratory experiments, that it was built out of the statistical patterns found in an observed stochastic dynamics, and that it was aimed at predicting the statistical distributions of that stochastic dynamics. The current formulation of quantum mechanics essentially encompasses a set of rules for obtaining the probabilities associated with the dynamics of quantum systems.

The theory does not state anything beyond that. A point that allowed many physicists to pragmatically take the theory as it is, not dwelling on the *why quantum systems work that way*, that is, to take the theory as a rule book that works, is robustly tested empirically, applying it to problems following what is usually called a *shut up and calculate stance*.

When one starts to ask on the *why quantum systems work that way*, the interpretations enter into play, but they go beyond the physical setting of the theory in the sense that they are related to ontological questions; that is, each interpretation regards the ontological issue of physical reality and why the quantum dynamics follows the *echoes* with probabilities coincident with the *echo intensities*.

In the pragmatic stance, one just takes the formalism as a recipe, calculates the *echo intensities* without dwelling further on it. Any result in quantum mechanics applying the formalism is valid and empirically testable and the formalism has time and again, during twentieth and twenty-first centuries, been shown to be robust in its predictions.

One way out of the ontological questioning would be to assume that we are dealing with human representations, that we cannot speak of a reality independent of human representations and experiments, that is, that the question of what reality really is outside those representations and experiments cannot be answered and, therefore, one just postulates that the field follows the *echoes*. This was the approach of the Copenhagen school, including Bohr and Born, leading to Born's rule that the probabilities are coincident with the *echoes*, a rule that is introduced, usually, in quantum mechanics' classes as a postulate, a very detailed description of this can be found in [7].

Contrasting with the Copenhagen school are the ontological schools, so called because they assume a reality independent of human representations and experiments.

Quantum mechanics itself does not state anything about this, so there is room for proposals; Cramer [7], for instance, considers these interpretations as actually new physical theories that go beyond the strict formalism and introduce new conjecture that cannot be tested under the formalism itself. The ontological interpretations that include the Bohmian and Everettian lines are all consistent with the formalism, that is, they agree with the formalism and mathematical methods of quantum mechanics and, therefore, cannot be tested using just the formalism.

In the case of Cramer, his proposed transactional interpretation (TI) of quantum mechanics [7] considers a probabilistic selection in terms of a *quantum handshake* (Cramer's transaction), where there is a sequential hierarchical selection for a quantum handshake linking the beginning and endpoint of the quantum dynamics, where each alternative is evaluated probabilistically for the formation of a quantum handshake or not; if no handshake is selected for a given alternative, the quantum dynamics proceeds to the next alternative. In each case, the probability for a quantum handshake is equal to the *echo* intensity, thus deriving Born's rule from within the formalism, instead of assuming it as a postulate.

Everett [8] assumed that all alternatives for a quantum system are actualized simultaneously in different cosmic branches. This led to the many worlds interpretation (MWI). MWI's proposal is, thus, that reality is multidimensional and the formalism is considered to be describing such a multidimensional reality that is a single Cosmos with many worlds (many branching lines). This conjecture cannot be tested empirically; it is consistent with the formalism and agrees with the predictions of quantum mechanics. Namely, the statistical measure associated with repeated experiments made on quantum systems tends to coincide with the *echo* intensities since the *echo intensities* coincide with the existence intensity of each world, recovering a statistical measure upon repeated experiments, as argued by Everett in [8] regarding Born's rule.

Bohm initially worked on the pilot wave model for quantum mechanics but just as a first approximation. Indeed, in [9], the author addressed the pilot wave model as a first approximation but then criticized it, in particular, in regard to the assumption of a particle being separate from the field; even more, in [9], Bohm defended that, at a lower level, the particle does not move as a permanently existing entity, but is formed in a random way by suitable concentrations of the field's energy. Furthermore, he considered that any quantum field was characterized by a nonlocal dynamics, and that the equations of quantum mechanics were just an approximation, an average that emerged at the quantum level, proposing the concept of quantum force and hypothesizing the existence of a subquantum level, so that both the quantum and subquantum levels play a fundamental role in the field's dynamics.

Gonçalves in [6] addressed the relation between the *echo* and Bohm's proposal recovering the Bohmian concept of quantum force [9, 10].

In this interpretation, the *echo* is associated with a dynamics of a quantum field for the evaluation of each alternative; the probing and response dynamics, thus, play a fundamental role, allowing a quantum field, any quantum field, to compute each alternative in parallel, leading to an *echo* associated with each alternative.

As argued in [6], the intensity (modulated) *echoes* would, thus, have a functional role as signalizers of an order to be risen (in the QUANN case, this *order* corresponds to a specific quantum neural firing pattern); the field's quantum and subquantum levels would, then, work in tandem, mobilizing the forces needed to make rise one specific alternative, and the resulting field lines of force, therefore, coincide, in their intensities, with the *echo intensities*.

This quantum computational dynamics, present in quantum mechanics' formalism, works as a basic form of *quantum "learning" dynamics*, where the quantum field "learns" about each alternative in the probe (forward propagating) and response (back propagating) dynamics and, then, the field's lines of force are formed along the *echoes* resulting from the encounters of matching probe and response vectors, with a force intensity that matches the corresponding *echo*'s intensity; the field then follows one of these lines of force with a probability that coincides with the *echo intensity*, so that the following of a given line of force is similar to a bifurcation dynamics where the field will follow, stochastically, one of the branches with a probability that coincides with the force intensity associated with each branch [6].

There is a consequence that comes from assuming the Bohmian framework, namely, from the Bohm's conjecture that a subquantum level randomness averages out at the quantum level, but may lead to small deviations from the theoretical probabilities [9, 10]; if such a conjecture holds, then deviations in quantum physical experiments with actual quantum computers may always take place, such that, even if we were to reduce the interaction with the environment to zero (or close to zero), we could still have deviations due to subquantum level fluctuations, so that the field would tend to follow the lines of force with probabilities that would hold on average but with some deviations that might occur in each case.

While Bohm's proposal is potentially testable, at the present stage of scientific and technological development, we have not yet found a way to test the subquantum proposal regarding quantum physical systems, and, in particular, to test, empirically, the possibility that deviations from the main lines of force that agree with a theory's prediction are not due to environmental noise and, rather, to subquantum level fluctuations.

All main interpretations, as reviewed above, agree with quantum mechanics' general predictions, even Bohm, who considers that the predictions will hold empirically on average, therefore, the interpretations do not have, at present, a direct consequence on the results of technological implementation of quantum computers, as long as one is not dealing with fundamental ontological issues regarding the computational nature of quantum fields, but rather with the technological application of quantum algorithms, one is free to choose any interpretation since it is consistent with the main formalism and results.

We consider, nonetheless, that future research directions on Bohm's conjectural line may prove fruitful both at a theoretical and technological level, concerning the issue of quantum errors. This point, however, goes beyond the current chapter's scope. The results that follow, as of any work using the formalism of quantum mechanics, hold for any interpretation of the theory. However, having made that point, we will return to Bohm's conjecture regarding some of the results obtained in the next section, regarding the issue of quantum computing errors.

3. Implementing quantum artificial neural networks on IBM's quantum computers

The development of quantum computing devices has opened up the possibility of transitioning from the purely theoretical approach to QUANNs to an experimental implementation of these networks. A particular example is IBM's quantum processors, available via cloud, under IBM Q Experience, using *superconducting transmon quantum processing units*.

The term *transmon* stands for *transmission-line shunted plasma oscillation*. A *transmon qubit* [11, 12] is an attempt at a technological implementation of a *qubit* for quantum computation, using superconductivity and Josephson junctions, gaining in charge noise insensitivity [11, 12]. The control, coupling, and measurement are implemented by means of microwave resonators and circuit quantum electrodynamics.

IBM has different *transmon*-based quantum computers in different locations around the world and provides access to these computers via cloud; this availability allows researchers to implement quantum experiments on actual quantum computers via cloud using IBM Q Experience, opening also the way for programmers to run algorithms on quantum computers by using the Python library Qiskit, which allows for the programmer to build quantum circuits in the Python code and manage the cloud-based access for simulation and experiments. The examples addressed in the present section all used Qiskit and two devices were employed: the "IBM Q 5 Tenerife" (ibmqx4)[2] and the "IBM Q 16 Melbourne"[3] (ibmq_16_melbourne).

The "IBM Q 5 Tenerife" device is a 5 *qubit* device with quantum registers labeled from Q0 to Q4, and the connectivity is, according to IBM, provided by two coplanar waveguide (CPW) resonators with resonances around 6.6 GHz (coupling Q2, Q3, and Q4) and 7.0 GHz (coupling Q0, Q1, and Q2).

The "IBM Q 16 Melbourne" device is a 14 *qubit* device with a connectivity that is, in turn, provided by a total of 22 CPW bus resonators each one connecting two quantum registers. For both the Tenerife and Melbourne devices, each quantum register also has a dedicated CPW readout resonator attached for control and readout.

From a computational model standpoint, we can treat the network connections and resulting quantum computing framework, provided by these physical devices, as a form of QUANN, where the conditional neural gates must obey the quantum device's basic topology in what regards the possible quantum controlled gates.

This is so because the quantum registers are linked in specific topologies that limit how conditional quantum operations are implemented; this is a main characteristic of QUANNs, namely, the conditional unitary gates implemented in neural computational circuits are dependent upon the topology and links between the different artificial neurons.

For the simplest algorithms, we can use just a few registers and connections, which means that each quantum device can simulate different QUANNs, within the restrictions of their respective topologies.

For a QUANN using all the quantum registers in the device, the types of algorithms are limited by the device structure, which can only implement a specific neural network topology and link direction.

In **Figures 1** and **2**, we, respectively, show the connectivity structure of the "IBM Q 5 Tenerife" and the "IBM Q 16 Melbourne" devices.

Having introduced the two devices, we now exemplify the theoretical and experimental implementation of a QUANN, on these devices, for a basic problem: the XOR Boolean function representation. This is a relevant example in the artificial neural network (ANN) literature, since the classical feedforward ANN needs a hidden layer to solve this problem, while its quantum counterpart does not [4].

Namely, a three-neuron QUANN with two input neurons feeding forward to a single output neuron is capable of representing the XOR function, while, in the classical case, we need an additional hidden layer comprised of two neurons. This is a feature of QUANNs that is generalizable to other Boolean functions as discussed in [4] regarding the computational efficiency of QUANNs over classical ANNs.

The reason for the greater efficiency is linked to entanglement, namely, the output neuron's firing dynamics can become entangled with the input layer's firing dynamics by way of the implementation of conditional NOT (CNOT) gates,

[2] The relevant elements on this processor, including the quantum circuit structure, can be consulted at the Qiskit backend website: https://github.com/Qiskit/qiskit-backend-information/tree/master/backends/tenerife/V1 (consulted in 21/10/2018)

[3] The relevant elements on this processor, including the quantum circuit structure, can be consulted at the Qiskit backend website: https://github.com/Qiskit/qiskit-backend-information/blob/master/backends/melbourne/V1/README.md (consulted in 21/10/2018).

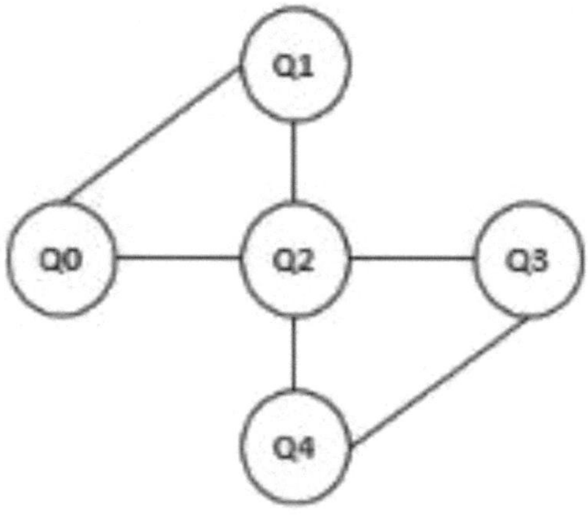

Figure 1.
IBM Q 5 Tenerife (ibmqx4) connectivity structure.

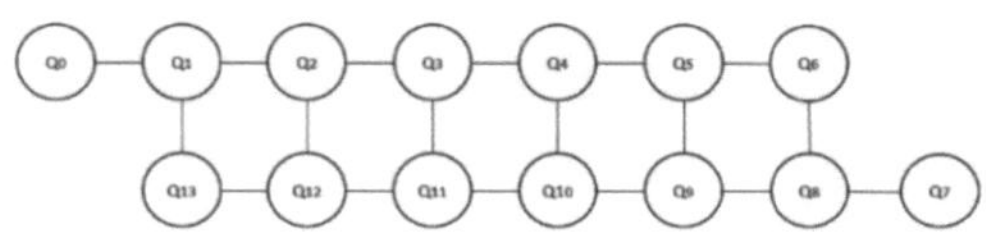

Figure 2.
IBM Q 16 Melbourne (ibmq_16_melbourne) connectivity structure.

providing for an example of the importance of entanglement in the efficiency of quantum computation over classical computation, a point that was object of detailed discussion in [4] regarding the relevance of entanglement for quantum neural computational efficiency.

3.1 The XOR representation problem

The XOR Boolean function representation problem is such that we want an output neuron to fire when the input neurons' firing patterns are reversed and to remain nonfiring when the input neurons' firing patterns are aligned. This means that the neural network's output follows the XOR truth table with the output neuron firing when the XOR function evaluates to "True" and not firing otherwise.

In this case, as shown in [4], the XOR function representation problem can be solved by a standard quantum feedforward neural network with no hidden layer, by taking advantage of quantum entanglement dynamics.

Formally, the quantum circuit, in the forward direction, can be represented by the following chain:

$$\hat{C} = \hat{U}_3 \hat{U}_2 \hat{U}_1 \tag{21}$$

with the gates, respectively, given by:

$$\hat{U}_1 = \hat{U}_{WH} \otimes \hat{U}_{WH} \otimes \hat{1} \tag{22}$$

$$\hat{U}_2 = |0\rangle\langle 0| \otimes \hat{1} \otimes \hat{1} + |1\rangle\langle 1| \otimes \hat{1} \otimes \hat{\sigma}_1 \tag{23}$$

$$\hat{U}_3 = \hat{1} \otimes |0\rangle\langle 0| \otimes \hat{1} + \hat{1} \otimes |1\rangle\langle 1| \otimes \hat{\sigma}_1 \tag{24}$$

We begin with all three neurons in a nonfiring dynamics; then, the propagation from input to output (in the forward direction of the computational circuit) yields:

$$\left\langle s_1s_2s_3\middle|\hat{C}\middle|000\right\rangle = \langle s_1s_2s_3|\hat{U}_3\,\hat{U}_2\hat{U}_1|000\rangle =$$
$$= \langle s_1s_2s_3|\hat{U}_3\hat{U}_2\left(\frac{|000\rangle + |010\rangle + |100\rangle + |110\rangle}{2}\right) =$$
$$= \langle s_1s_2s_3|\hat{U}_3\left(\frac{|000\rangle + |010\rangle + |101\rangle + |111\rangle}{2}\right) =$$
$$= \langle s_1s_2s_3|\left(\frac{|000\rangle + |011\rangle + |101\rangle + |110\rangle}{2}\right) =$$
$$= \frac{\delta_{s_1,0}\delta_{s_2,0}\delta_{s_3,0}}{2} + \frac{\delta_{s_1,0}\delta_{s_2,1}\delta_{s_3,1}}{2} + \frac{\delta_{s_1,1}\delta_{s_2,0}\delta_{s_3,1}}{2} + \frac{\delta_{s_1,1}\delta_{s_2,1}\delta_{s_3,0}}{2} \tag{25}$$

The result in Eq. (25) means that the only probed final alternatives are those where the XOR rule $s_3 = s_1 \oplus s_2$ holds; that is, these are the only alternatives where there is a nonzero amplitude.

Likewise, back propagation from the output to the input yields the same result, that is, the only responses come from outputs where the XOR rule $s_3 = s_1 \oplus s_2$ holds, as the following derivation shows:

$$\left\langle 000\middle|\hat{C}^\dagger\middle|s_1s_2s_3\right\rangle = \langle 000|\hat{U}_1{}^\dagger\,\hat{U}_2{}^\dagger\hat{U}_3{}^\dagger|s_1s_2s_3\rangle =$$
$$= \delta_{s_2,0}\langle 000|\hat{U}_1{}^\dagger\hat{U}_2{}^\dagger|s_1s_2s_3\rangle + \delta_{s_2,1}\langle 000|\hat{U}_1{}^\dagger\hat{U}_2{}^\dagger|s_1s_21-s_3\rangle =$$
$$= \delta_{s_1,0}\delta_{s_2,0}\langle 000|\hat{U}_1{}^\dagger|s_1s_2s_3\rangle + \delta_{s_1,0}\delta_{s_2,1}\langle 000|\hat{U}_1{}^\dagger|s_1s_21-s_3\rangle +$$
$$+\delta_{s_1,1}\delta_{s_2,0}\langle 000|\hat{U}_1{}^\dagger|s_1s_21-s_3\rangle + \delta_{s_1,1}\delta_{s_2,1}\langle 000|\hat{U}_1{}^\dagger|s_1s_2s_3\rangle =$$
$$= \frac{\delta_{s_1,0}\delta_{s_2,0}\delta_{s_3,0}}{2} + \frac{\delta_{s_1,0}\delta_{s_2,1}\delta_{s_3,1}}{2} + \frac{\delta_{s_1,1}\delta_{s_2,0}\delta_{s_3,1}}{2} + \frac{\delta_{s_1,1}\delta_{s_2,1}\delta_{s_3,0}}{2} \tag{26}$$

Replacing Eqs. (25) and (26) in the general Eq. (17) yields, for this quantum circuit, the *echo intensities*:

$$\langle s_1s_2s_3|\hat{\rho}_{out}|s_1s_2s_3\rangle = \left\langle s_1s_2s_3\middle|\hat{C}\middle|000\right\rangle\left\langle 000\middle|\hat{C}^\dagger\middle|s_1s_2s_3\right\rangle = \frac{\delta_{s_3,s_1\oplus s_2}}{4} \tag{27}$$

That is, the forward and back propagation is such that the *echoes* are only formed for the cases where the rule $s_3 = s_1 \oplus s_2$ holds, leading to a ¼ probability associated with each alternative firing pattern of the first two neurons.

The **Figure 3** shows the theoretical results from the above equations, the simulation in the IBM quantum assembly language (QASM) simulator and the experimental implementation on the Tenerife (ibmqx4) and Melbourne (ibmq_16_melbourne) devices.

The QASM simulation expresses, as expected, the basic random results from the repeated experiments, which is associated with the fundamental stochastic dynamics underlying quantum processing; however, the simulator results agree with the theoretical results, so that the basic XOR computation holds, that is, in each case, the output neuron exhibits the firing pattern that is consistent with the XOR rule.

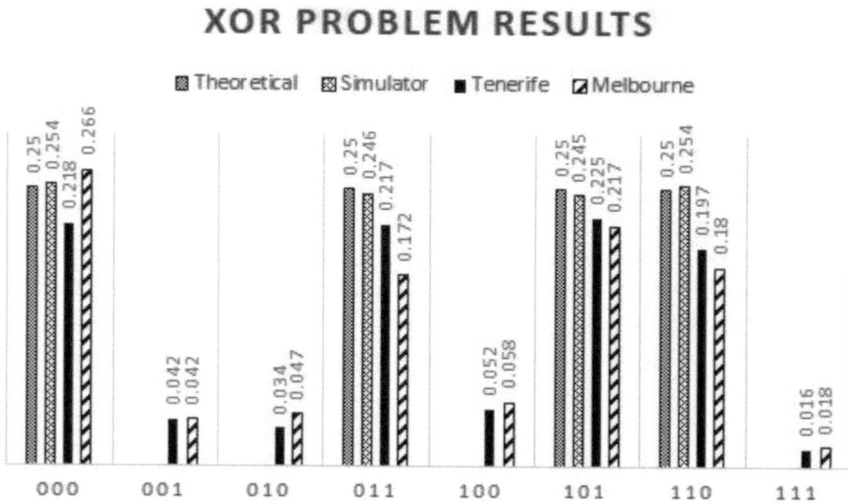

Figure 3.
Theoretical and experimental implementation of the XOR representation problem on the QASM simulator, Tenerife and Melbourne devices, with 8192 shots.

In the case of experiments, the XOR rule is predominant, that is, the dominant frequencies are those consistent with the circuit; there are, however, also a few residual cases that deviate from the XOR rule, all with low relative frequencies. These deviations are to be expected on the actual physical devices. For the Tenerife device, the relative frequency of cases that follow the XOR rule is 0.857; for the Melbourne device, this relative frequency is 0.835.

One of the main problems in physical implementation of quantum computation is the presence of errors. Indeed, the equations are derived for an isolated circuit so that the only *echoes* are those matching the quantum circuit; therefore, in an isolated QUANN, the stochastic results from repeated trials tend, in a frequentist approach, to the actual probabilities with zero frequencies associated with the alternatives for which no *echo* is produced. This is a basic property of quantum mechanics as predicted by the theory, and explains that the QASM simulator gets a zero measure for those alternatives for which there is no *echo*.

Of course, if Bohm's conjecture regarding the subquantum dynamics [9, 10] is right, then, even for a sufficiently isolated circuit, small deviations coming from the subquantum level may be present and lead to *echoes* that do not correspond to those of the main computing circuit. In any other interpretation that does not assume a subquantum dynamics and that takes the formalism to be exact, then, such deviations, for an isolated system, are considered physically impossible.

While we cannot rule out Bohm's subquantum hypothesis, we cannot also confirm it for now, since one never has a completely isolated circuit, and both conjectural lines (Bohmian and others) agree that some deviations on physical devices will always be present due to the environment.

The differences between the two conjectural lines, for quantum computer science, are worth considering regarding quantum error correction; however, for now, in regard to the technological issue of quantum error correction, we cannot yet make use of Bohm's conjecture that the quantum probabilities are average quantities and that subquantum fluctuations may introduce small deviations that average out at the quantum level to lead to the main experimental agreement with the theory.

Having provided, through the XOR problem, an example of how quantum neural computation can be run experimentally on IBM's quantum devices, we now address artificial intelligence (AI) applications; we are interested in the theoretical and experimental implementation of a form of reinforcement learning using QUANNs, namely the quantum neural reinforcement learning (QNRL) and its connection to quantum robotics and quantum adaptive computation.

3.2 Quantum neural reinforcement learning, robotics, and quantum adaptive computation

Quantum robotics involves the need for the development of quantum adaptive algorithms that allow the robot to process alternatives and select appropriate actions using quantum rules [6, 13–15], that is, to incorporate decisions in quantum AI. In this context, there are two major types of artificial agents that one may consider:

- classical agents that implement classical actions but whose cognitive substrate is quantum computational;
- quantum agents that implement quantum operations on a quantum target.

The first type of agent is addressed as a classical robot dealing with problems at a classical level but whose computational substrate is run via cloud access on a quantum computer, thus, pointing toward a possible future where quantum computation is incorporated on different robotic systems by way of the internet of things and cloud-based access to quantum devices.

The second type of agents corresponds to *quantum software robots* (*quantum bots*) that are implemented within a quantum computer and can be used for the adaptive management of target quantum registers and for the purpose of more complex adaptive computation [6, 13–15].

This second type of agents forms the basis for AI solutions aiming at intelligent quantum computing systems with application in quantum internet technologies and, also, possible quantum adaptive error correction.

This latter point (quantum adaptive error correction) must draw specifically on the empirical implementation in physical devices, since it is this implementation that may ultimately test the best adaptive algorithms for quantum error correction. A basic direction, in this case, regards *echo* strengthening, in order to diminish the *echoes* coming from alternatives that do not fall in an intended computation.

We do not address this last point here, but rather illustrate the implementation of the first type of agent in the context of an adaptive computation of a classical gamble, namely, optimal action selection in a classical gambling problem through quantum neural reinforcement learning (QNRL).

In this case, the artificial agent is dealing with a classical problem and implementing its decision processing on a QUANN, namely, the agent has an action set described by 2^d binary strings; following an evolutionary computation framework, we use d-length genetic codes to address actions, so that the actions' codes are comprised of d loci, each with two alleles, 0 and 1.

Now, given each alternative action, the agent is offered a classical gamble on a measurable space $(\Omega, \wp)$ where $\wp$ is a sigma-algebra of subsets of Ω and $\Omega = \{w_0, w_1, \ldots, w_{N-1}\}$ is the set of rewards for the gamble, which we consider, in this example, to be discrete, although the results also apply to continuous reward spaces and (classical) probability distributions.

Now, for each action genetic code $\mathbf{s} \in \mathrm{A}_2^d$ there is a corresponding gamble probability measure $P_\mathbf{s}$ that is offered to the agent, so that the conditional expected value for the reward w can be calculated as:

$$E[w|\mathbf{s}] = \sum_{n=0}^{N-1} w_n P_{\mathbf{s}}[w_n] \tag{28}$$

The goal for the agent is to select the action that maximizes this conditional expected reward, that is:

$$\mathbf{s}^* = \arg\max_{\mathbf{s}} E[w|\mathbf{s}] \tag{29}$$

To solve the optimization problem in Eq. (29), we use a variant of QNRL, which applies modular networked learning [16], in the sense that, instead of a single neural network for a single problem, we expand the cognitive architecture and work with a modular system of neural networks.

Modular networked learning (MNL) was addressed in [16] and applied to financial market prediction, where, instead of a single problem and a single target, one uses an expanded cognitive architecture to work on multiple targets with a module assigned to each target and possible links between the modules used to map links between subproblems of a more complex problem.

For modular neural networks, the resulting cognitive architecture resembles an artificial brain with specialized "brain regions" devoted to different tasks and connections between different neural modules corresponding to connections between different brain regions. In the present case, the agent's "artificial brain" (as shown in **Figure 4**) is comprised of three "brain regions" connected with each other for a specific functionality, where the first module (first brain region) corresponds to the action exploration region, the second module (second brain region) corresponds to the reward processing region, and the third module to the decision region.

The connections between the modules follow the hierarchical process associated with the necessary quantum reinforcement learning for each action, **Figure 4** expresses this relation. The reinforcement learning, in this case, is a form of quantum search, implemented on the above modular structure, that proceeds in two stages: the exploration stage and the exploitation stage.

In the exploration stage, the agent's first brain region, taking advantage of quantum superposition, explores with equal weights, in parallel, each alternative initial action and the second brain region processes the conditional expected rewards; this last processing is based on optimizing quantum circuits [6], where

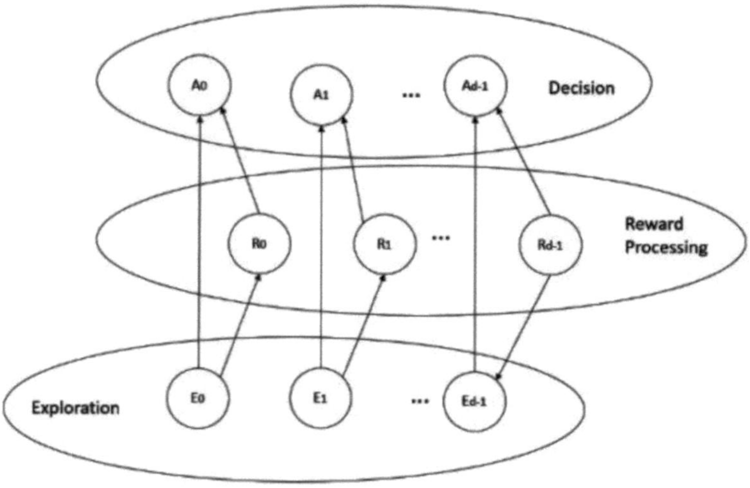

Figure 4.
Modular structure for the reward maximization problem.

the unitary operator for the second brain region incorporates the optimization itself.

The second brain region will work as a form of oracle in the remaining adaptive computation and allows for the agent's artificial brain to implement an optimal expected reward-seeking dynamics.

Now, in the second phase of the exploration stage, the synaptic connections from the first to the second brain region are activated, leading to a quantum entangled dynamics between the two brain regions, where the first region acts as the control (input layer) and the second as the target (output layer).

Thus, at the end of the exploration stage, the first two brain regions exhibit an entangled dynamics. This is a basic point of quantum strategic cognition, in the sense that the processing of the alternative courses of action is not localized in a specific neuron or neurons, but rather it leads to quantum correlations between different brain regions; these connections allow the artificial brain to efficiently select the best course of action, from the evaluation of the alternatives and rewards.

In the exploitation stage, the synaptic connections from the first brain region (the action exploration region) to the third brain region (the decision region) are activated first, so that the decision region is first processing the explored alternative actions, becoming entangled with the action exploration region; then, the synaptic connections between the reward processing region and the decision region are activated for the conditional expected reward processing by the decision module. In this way, the decision module makes the transition for the optimal action, consulting the "oracle" (which is the reward processing module) only once.

The artificial brain thus takes advantage of quantum entanglement in order to adaptively output the optimal action. Formalizing this dynamics, the artificial brain is initialized in a nonfiring probe and response dynamics so that the initial density is:

$$\hat{\rho}_0 = |0\rangle\langle 0|^{\otimes 3d} \tag{30}$$

Now, we denote by $\mathbf{s}_k^*$ the *k-th* bit in the string $\mathbf{s}^*$, and use the following notation for the maximization in Eq. (29) evaluated at the *k-th* bit:

$$\mathbf{s}_k^* = \arg\max_{\mathbf{s},\, k} E[w|\mathbf{s}] \tag{31}$$

Using this notation, the first phase of the exploration stage is given by the unitary operator:

$$\hat{U}_1 = \\ = \hat{U}_{WH}{}^{\otimes d} \otimes_{k=1}^{d} \left(\cos\left(\frac{\arg\max_{\mathbf{s},\, k} E[w|\mathbf{s}]}{2} \pi \right) \hat{1} - i \sin\left(\frac{\arg\max_{\mathbf{s},\, k} E[w|\mathbf{s}]}{2} \pi \right) \hat{\sigma}_2 \right) \otimes \hat{1}^{\otimes d} \tag{32}$$

The operator incorporates the optimization dynamics into the conditional quantum gates' parameters themselves. Since we have:

$$\left(\cos\left(\frac{\arg\max_{\mathbf{s},\, k} E[w|\mathbf{s}]}{2} \pi \right) \hat{1} - i \sin\left(\frac{\arg\max_{\mathbf{s},\, k} E[w|\mathbf{s}]}{2} \pi \right) \hat{\sigma}_2 \right) |0\rangle \tag{33}$$

$$= \cos\left(\frac{\underset{\mathbf{s},\,k}{\arg\max}\, E[w|\mathbf{s}]}{2}\pi\right)|0\rangle + \sin\left(\frac{\underset{\mathbf{s},\,k}{\arg\max}\, E[w|\mathbf{s}]}{2}\pi\right)|1\rangle = |\mathbf{s}_k^*\rangle$$

after the first phase of the of exploration stage, the resulting density is given by:

$$\hat{\rho}_1 = \hat{U}_1\hat{\rho}_0\hat{U}_1^{\dagger} = |+\rangle\langle+|^{\otimes d} \otimes |\mathbf{s}^*\rangle\langle\mathbf{s}^*| \otimes |0\rangle\langle 0|^{\otimes d} \tag{34}$$

Thus, the neural field is probing, for the first brain region, each alternative neural pattern (each alternative action) with equal weight, the response dynamics also comes, for the first brain region, from each alternative neural pattern with equal weight, which means that the *echoes* for the first brain region are independent from the *echoes* for the remaining brain regions and show an equal intensity associated with each alternative neural pattern.

On the other hand, for the second brain region, the neural field exhibits a reward-seeking dynamics that is adaptive with respect to the optimal action; that is, the probing dynamics is directed toward the optimal action and the response dynamics also comes from the optimal action, so that, due to the adaptive unitary propagation, the second brain region is projecting over the optimum value, and this is the only *echo* that it gets.

The third brain region still has a projective dynamics toward the nonfiring neural activity.

Now, for the second phase of the exploration stage, we have the operator:

$$\hat{U}_2 = \left[\sum_{\mathbf{s}\in A_2^d} |\mathbf{s}\rangle\langle\mathbf{s}| \otimes_{k=1}^{d}\left((1-s_k)\hat{1} + s_k\hat{\sigma}_1\right)\right] \otimes \hat{1}^{\otimes d} \tag{35}$$

which leads to the density after the second phase of the exploration stage:

$$\hat{\rho}_2 = \hat{U}_2\hat{\rho}_1\hat{U}_2^{\dagger} = \sum_{\mathbf{r},\,\mathbf{s}\in A_2^d} \frac{|\mathbf{r}\rangle\langle\mathbf{s}| \otimes_{k=1}^{d} |\mathbf{s}_k^* \oplus r_k\rangle\langle\mathbf{s}_k^* \oplus s_k|}{2^d} \otimes |0\rangle\langle 0|^{\otimes d} \tag{36}$$

Thus, after the second phase, the first and second brain regions exhibit an entangled probe and response dynamics, where the neural field, for second brain region, is effectively computing both the rewards and the explored actions.

Next comes the exploitation stage with the neural processing for the decision module (the third brain region).

The first step of the exploitation stage is the processing of the initially explored actions, by way of the operator:

$$\hat{U}_3 = \sum_{\mathbf{s}\in A_2^d} |\mathbf{s}\rangle\langle\mathbf{s}| \otimes \hat{1}^{\otimes d} \otimes_{k=1}^{d}\left((1-s_k)\hat{1} + s_k\hat{\sigma}_1\right) \tag{37}$$

which leads to the density:

$$\hat{\rho}_3 = \hat{U}_3\hat{\rho}_2\hat{U}_3^{\dagger} = \sum_{\mathbf{r},\,\mathbf{s}\in A_2^d} \frac{|\mathbf{r}\rangle\langle\mathbf{s}| \otimes_{k=1}^{d} |\mathbf{s}_k^* \oplus r_k\rangle\langle\mathbf{s}_k^* \oplus s_k| \otimes |\mathbf{r}\rangle\langle\mathbf{s}|}{2^d} \tag{38}$$

That is, the probe and response dynamics for the third brain region are correlated and coincident with the probe and response dynamics for the first brain region, so that the third brain region is effectively computing the initially explored actions.

Now, the second step for the third brain region results from the activation of the synaptic links with the second brain region, leading to the conditional unitary operator:

$$\hat{U}_4 = \sum_{\mathbf{s} \in \mathrm{A}_2^d} \hat{1}^{\otimes d} \otimes |\mathbf{s}\rangle\langle\mathbf{s}| \otimes_{k=1}^{d} \left((1 - s_k)\hat{1} + s_k \hat{\sigma}_1\right) \tag{39}$$

Under this operator, we get the final density:

$$\hat{\rho}_4 = \hat{U}_4 \hat{\rho}_3 \hat{U}_4^{\dagger} = = \sum_{\mathbf{r},\, \mathbf{s} \in \mathrm{A}_2^d} \frac{|\mathbf{r}\rangle\langle\mathbf{s}| \otimes_{k=1}^{d} \left(\left|\mathbf{s}_k^* \oplus r_k\right\rangle\left\langle\mathbf{s}_k^* \oplus s_k\right| \otimes \left|r_k \oplus \left(\mathbf{s}_k^* \oplus r_k\right)\right\rangle\left\langle s_k \oplus \left(\mathbf{s}_k^* \oplus s_k\right)\right|\right)}{2^d} \tag{40}$$

Since we have the Boolean equality $p \oplus (q \oplus p) = q$, this means that the above density can be simplified, so that the neural field's probe and response dynamics for the third brain region projects over the optimal action:

$$\hat{\rho}_4 = \hat{U}_4 \hat{\rho}_3 \hat{U}_4^{\dagger} = \left(\sum_{\mathbf{r},\, \mathbf{s} \in \mathrm{A}_2^d} \frac{|\mathbf{r}\rangle\langle\mathbf{s}| \otimes_{k=1}^{d} \left|\mathbf{s}_k^* \oplus r_k\right\rangle\left\langle\mathbf{s}_k^* \oplus s_k\right|}{2^d} \right) \otimes |\mathbf{s}^*\rangle\langle\mathbf{s}^*| \tag{41}$$

The third brain region's computation takes advantage of the entangled dynamics between the first and second brain regions to learn the optimal action. For the final density, while the first and second brain regions exhibit an entangled probe and response dynamics, the third brain region is always projecting over the optimum.

It is important to stress how QNRL takes advantage of quantum entanglement such that the neural field for the third brain region followed each alternative action and then the reward processing dynamics to find the optimum in all these alternative paths, so that the optimal action is always followed by the agent.

As an example of the above problem, let us consider the case where we the reward set is $\Omega = \{-1, 1\}$, and that there are two possible actions 0 and 1 leading, respectively, to the classical probability measures P_0 and P_1, with $P_0[w = 1] = 0.4$ and $P_1[w = 1] = 0.6$; then, we get the probabilities of selection for each gamble and device shown in **Table 1**, for 8192 repeated experiments.

As expected, the QASM simulator always selects the action 1, which is the best performing action by the conditional expected payoff criterion. The Tenerife device selects the correct action with a proportion of 0.778, while the Melbourne device selects the correct action with a proportion of 0.647. If, instead of the above gamble profile, we had $P_0[w = 1] = 0.6$ and $P_1[w = 1] = 0.4$, the optimal choice would be the action 0; in this case, as shown in **Table 2**, the QASM simulator, again, selects the correct action each time. The Tenerife device, in turn, selects the correct action with a 0.857 frequency and the Melbourne device with a 0.814 frequency.

In **Figure 5**, we show the Melbourne device's results[4] when we have four actions for the same rewards profile, and the probabilities are $P_{00}[w = 1] = 0.6$, $P_{01}[w = 1] = 0.4$, $P_{10}[w = 1] = 0.8$, and $P_{11}[w = 1] = 0.9$, still setting the *rewards* to $\Omega = \{-1, 1\}$.

In this case, if we run the experiment on the QASM backend, with 8192 shots, we get the action encoded by the string 11 with relative frequency equal to 1, which

[4] We can only use the Melbourne device since the Tenerife device does not have the required capacity in terms of number of quantum registers.

Device	Action	
	0	**1**
QASM	0	1
Tenerife	0.222	0.778
Melbourne	0.353	0.647

Table 1.
Results for two alternative actions using the QASM simulator, the Tenerife device (ibmqx4) and the Melbourne device (ibmq_16_melbourne); in each case, 8192 shots were used, with $P_0[w = 1] = 0.4$ and $P_1[w = 1] = 0.6$.

Device	Action	
	0	**1**
QASM	1	0
Tenerife	0.857	0.143
Melbourne	0.814	0.186

Table 2.
Results for two actions using the QASM simulator, the Tenerife device (ibmqx4) and the Melbourne device (ibmq_16_melbourne); in each case, 8192 shots were used, with $P_0[w = 1] = 0.6$ and $P_1[w = 1] = 0.4$.

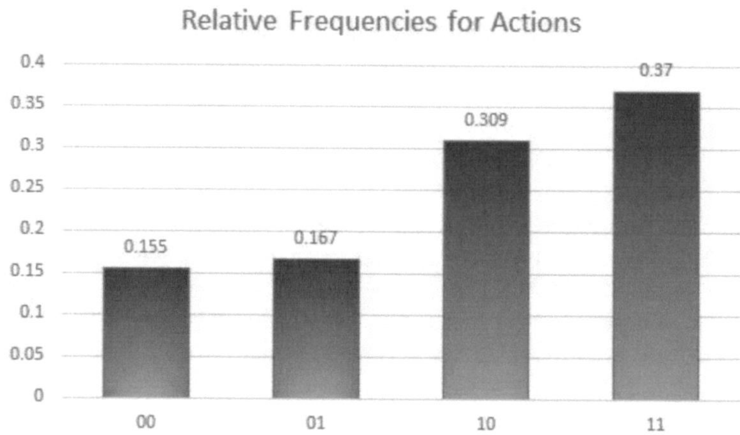

Figure 5.
Results for four actions using the Melbourne device ("ibmq_16_melbourne"), with 8192 shots used, and probability profiles given by: $P_{00}[w = 1] = 0.6$, $P_{01}[w = 1] = 0.4$, $P_{10}[w = 1] = 0.8$ and $P_{11}[w = 1] = 0.9$.

is the optimal action. If we run the experiment with the same number of shots on the Melbourne device, then, as shown in **Figure 5**, the output 11 is still the dominant action, however, with a proportion of 0.370, the second dominant action being non-residual and with a value of 0.309 occurs for the output 10.

Therefore, the first *qubit* tends to be measured with the right pattern with a proportion of 0.679 (0.309 + 0.370); the probability of the second *qubit* being correct given that the first is correct is only about 0.54492 (0.370/0.679). This suggests that the deviation may be due to the entanglement with the environment significantly deviating the second *qubit* from the correct pattern.

The above algorithm was implemented using Qiskit and Python's Object Oriented Programming (OOP); the code, shown in the appendix, exemplifies how OOP can be integrated with quantum computation for implementing quantum AI on any terminal, due to the cloud access to IBM's quantum resources, constituting an example of Quantum Object Oriented Programming (QOOP) using Qiskit.

The code defines the class "Agent" with an attribute that is the quantum neural network; in this case, the attribute will be assigned a quantum circuit with the required quantum and classical registers.

There are two methods that any instance of the class Agent must be able to implement: the first method manages the cloud access to IBM's resources, the second method implements the action selection and the quantum algorithm.

The inputs for the first method are the accounts to be loaded, for the classical computer to be able to access quantum computer via the cloud service, and the backend code, which, by default, is set to the QASM simulator but can be changed to any of the devices. The method returns the backend to be used.

The second method, for the action selection, has a structure that is specific to the problem in question; that is, the agent is offered a set of rewards and probabilities associated with each alternative action, and must choose the action that maximizes the conditional expected reward.

Thus, the probabilities are known to the agent and form part of the gamble that is offered to it; therefore, we are dealing with a decision problem under risk, and wish to address how the agent's QUANN can exhibit an adaptive computation with respect to this problem.

While, in the above equations, the adaptive nature of the quantum neural circuit was introduced in the unitary operator's parameters themselves, the Python code for the method must use the gamble's inputs to make the quantum circuit adaptive; that is, the method must be such that the agent designs its own cognitive architecture (updating its qnnet attribute) and quantum circuit using the inputs to the method, and, then, the agent must implement the cloud-based access to run, in IBM's quantum computers, the corresponding quantum algorithm.

The inputs for the method are, then, given by a list of probability distributions, where each line corresponds to a different probability gamble profile associated with each action, for instance, in the case of **Table 1**, the distributions are given by ([0.6, 0.4],[0.4, 0.6]). In the case of **Tables 1** and **2** and **Figure 5**, the rewards list is $[-1, 1]$.

The other two inputs for the method are the backend used which allows the agent that is instantiated in a classical computer to access via cloud the quantum computer, using the backend code (backend_used) and repeatedly running the algorithm on the respective device for a number of shots (num_shots).

The choose_action method's step zero is the extraction of the expected values and of the corresponding parameters for the adaptive gates, namely, the expected values array associated with each action is extracted by the agent using the Python library NumPy's dot product applied to the distributions and rewards lists.

The number of actions and dimension d that determines the network size are extracted from the length of the expected values array; then, the parameters for the adaptive gates are extracted by applying NumPy's argmax function on the expected values array and then converting the resulting index in binary format (using NumPy's binary_repr). Since the indexes match the lexicographic order of binary strings, the agent, thus, effectively extracts the parameters for the adaptive unitary gates.

Now, the next step is to set up the QUANN, including the three modules, the classical registers for the measurement of the final actions to be chosen and updating the agent's qnnet attribute, assigning it the corresponding Qiskit's quantum circuit object.

The last step implements the QNRL algorithm, following the inter-module links as per the main equations introduced in this section, and defines the quantum measurement for the decision module, executing the algorithm on the backend (taking advantage of the cloud access) and plotting the histogram to extract the main experimental relative frequencies obtained from the repeated experiments (the number of shots).

4. Conclusions

Cloud-based access to quantum computers opens up a major point: the empirical testing of algorithms and the implementation of computer programs in a quantum computational substrate has become feasible.

The IBM Q Experience constitutes an example of how a programmer can use Python programming language and IBM's Python Qiskit package for building programs that use quantum computation, limited only by the specific device resources, namely the number of quantum registers available.

For quantum AI and machine learning, this provides a way to effectively bring the algorithms from the theoretical level to the test level, allowing one to *test drive* different quantum AI frameworks on actual quantum computers. The work developed in the previous sections allowed us to provide several examples of such an implementation, with a few main points standing out:

- We showed how one can address IBM's superconducting *transmon devices* as examples of QUANNs, since, just as in a QUANN, the *devices* can only implement the conditional gates depending on the network topology and the directions of the links, which only allow for specific conditional gates to be implemented; as an example, the Tenerife device is a *bowtie feedforward network*, we cannot turn it into a recurrent network so that the gates have to be implemented following specific directions of the links (this limit can be experienced by any user that accesses the online resources and tries to visually build circuits in IBM Q Experience homepage).

- We exemplified how basic Boolean functions' representation, in this case the XOR function, can be implemented on a (physical) quantum computer using the cloud access to Tenerife and Melbourne devices and compared the experimental results with the theoretical derivation; a relevant point of this is that we only needed three quantum registers and no hidden layer to solve the XOR problem, a point already raised about this function and generalized to other functions in [4], regarding the theoretical efficiency of QUANNs.

- We addressed how a form of quantum adaptive computation, incorporating a reward-seeking behavior and a variant of QNRL, can be implemented, in the context of quantum robotics and AI, on different quantum devices.

The three main points above help strengthen two core arguments: the first is that quantum machine learning can now be tested on actual quantum computers, making it feasible to empirically test the algorithms; the second is that, in the near future, with further advancements in quantum computation and quantum hardware, quantum adaptive computation may be implemented on actual robots with a quantum cognitive architecture that is based on cloud access to a quantum computer.

The present work addresses both core arguments by exemplifying how a form of QNRL can be employed to implement quantum adaptive computation on a physical QUANN with cloud-based access, employing QOOP and addressing, experimentally, a decision under risk problem.

A. Python Code for Quantum Neural Reinforcement Learning Problem.

```
# Import NumPy and Qiskit's main functionalities
import numpy as np
from qiskit import ClassicalRegister, QuantumRegister, QuantumCircuit
from qiskit import execute
from qiskit import IBMQ
from qiskit.tools.visualization import plot_histogram
class Agent:
def __init__(self, qnnet):
self.qnnet = qnnet # agent's Quantum Neural Network
def get_backend(self,
load_accounts = True, # if accounts are to be loaded
backend_code = 'ibmq_qasm_simulator' # backend code
):
# Load IBM account if needed
if load_accounts == True:
IBMQ.load_accounts()
# Get the backend to use in the computation
backend_used = IBMQ.get_backend(backend_code)
# If one is not using the QASM simulator get the backend status
if backend_code! = 'ibmq_qasm_simulator':
print(backend_used.status())
# Return the backend used
return backend_used
def choose_action(self,
distributions, # probability distributions
rewards, # reward system
backend_used, # backed to be used
num_shots): # number of shots to run in quantum computer
# Step 0: get the expected values and unitary parameters:
# Get the expected values
expected_values = np.dot(distributions,rewards)
# Get the number of actions involved
num_actions = len(expected_values)
# Get the base number that we will need for the network size
dim = int.(np.log2(num_actions))
# Get the parameters for the adaptive gate
maxstring = np.binary_repr(np.argmax(expected_values), width = dim)
# Step 1: Setup the Quantum Artificial Neural Network:
# Get the number of quantum registers
q = QuantumRegister(3*dim)
# Get the number of classical registers
c = ClassicalRegister(dim)
# Setup the quantum neural network
self.qnnet = QuantumCircuit(q, c)
# Step 2: Implement the Reinforcement Learning Algorithm:
# Exploration Stage
for i in range(0,dim):
self.qnnet.h(q[i])
for j in range(0,dim):
self.qnnet.u3(float(maxstring[j])*np.pi,0,0,q[dim+j])
for k in range(0,dim):
```

```
self.qnnet.cx(q[k],q[dim+k])
# Exploitation Stage
for l in range(0,dim):
self.qnnet.cx(q[l],q[2*dim+l])
self.qnnet.cx(q[dim+l],q[2*dim+l])
# Quantum Measurement
for m in range(0,dim):
self.qnnet.measure(q[2*dim+m], c[dim-1-m])
# Execute the algorithm on the backend
job_exp = execute(self.qnnet, backend = backend_used, shots = num_shots)
# Plot the histogram
plot_histogram(job_exp.result().get_counts(self.qnnet))
```

Author details

Carlos Pedro dos Santos Gonçalves
University of Lisbon, Institute of Social and Political Sciences, Lisbon, Portugal

*Address all correspondence to: cgoncalves@iscsp.ulisboa.pt

References

[1] Menneer T. Quantum artificial neural networks [thesis]. Exeter: The University of Exeter; 1998

[2] Narayanan A, Meneer T. Quantum artificial neural network architectures and components. Information Sciences. 2000;**128**:231-255. DOI: 10.1016/S0020-0255(00)00055-4

[3] Schuld M, Sinayskiy I, Petruccione F. The quest for a quantum neural network. Quantum Information Processing. 2014;**13**(11):2567-2586. DOI: 10.1007/s11128-014-0809-8

[4] Gonçalves CP. Quantum cybernetics and complex quantum systems science: A quantum connectionist exploration. NeuroQuantology. 2015;**13**(1):35-48. DOI: 10.14704/nq.2015.13.1.804

[5] Gonçalves CP. Quantum neural machine learning: Backpropagation and dynamics. NeuroQuantology. 2017; **15**(1):22-41. DOI: 10.14704/nq.2017.15.1.1008

[6] Gonçalves CP. Quantum robotics, neural networks and the quantum force interpretation. NeuroQuantology. ISSN: 1303 5150

[7] Cramer JG. The Quantum Handshake: Entanglement, Nonlocality and Transactions. Cham: Springer. p. 218. DOI: 978-3-319-24640-6

[8] Everett H. Relative state' formulation of quantum mechanics. Reviews of Modern Physics. 1957;**29**(3):454-462. DOI: doi.org/10.1103/RevModPhys.29.454

[9] Bohm D. Causality and Chance in Modern Physics. London: Routledge; 1997 [1957]. p. 189. ISBN: 0-415-17440-6

[10] Bohm D, Hiley BJ. The Undivided Universe. New York: Routledge; 1995. p. 409. ISBN: 978-0415121859

[11] Koch J, Yu TM, Gambetta J, Houck AA, Schuster DI, Majer J, et al. Charge-insensitive qubit design derived from the Cooper pair box. Physical Review A. 2007;**76**:042319. DOI: 10.1103/PhysRevA.76.042319

[12] Schreier JA, Houck AA, Koch J, Schuster DI, Johnson BR, Chow JM, et al. Suppressing charge noise decoherence in superconducting charge qubits. Physical Review B;**77**:180502(R). DOI: 10.1103/PhysRevB.77.180502

[13] Benioff P. Quantum robots and environments. Physical Review A. 1998; **58**(2):893-904. DOI: 10.1103/PhysRevA.58.893

[14] Benioff P. Some foundational aspects of quantum computers and quantum robots. Superlattices and Microstructures. 1998;**23**(3–4):407-417. DOI: 10.1006/spmi.1997.0519

[15] Dong D-Y, Chen C-L, Zhang C-B, Chen Z-H. Quantum robot: Structure, algorithms and applications. Robotica. 2006;**24**(4):513-521. DOI: 10.1017/S0263574705002596

[16] Gonçalves CP. Financial Risk and Returns Prediction with Modular Networked Learning. arXiv: 1806.05876 [cs.LG]. 2018. Available from: https://arxiv.org/pdf/1806.05876.pdf [Accessed: 28-10-2018]

Chapter 6

Using Artificial Intelligence and Big Data-Based Documents to Optimize Medical Coding

Joseph Noussa-Yao, Didier Heudes and Patrice Degoulet

Abstract

Clinical information systems (CISs) in some hospitals streamline the data management from data warehouses. These warehouses contain heterogeneous information from all medical specialties that offer patient care services. It is increasingly difficult to manage large volumes of data in a specific clinical context such as quality coding of medical services. The document-based not only SQL (NoSQL) model can provide an accessible, extensive, and robust coding data management framework while maintaining certain flexibility. This paper focuses on the design and implementation of a big data-coding warehouse, and it also defines the rules to convert a conceptual model of coding into a document-oriented logical model. Using that model, we implemented and analyzed a big data-coding warehouse via the MongoDB database and evaluated it using data research mono- and multi-criteria and then calculated the precision of our model.

Keywords: diagnostic coding, clinical decision support, decision-making, big data, optimization, medical diagnostic computing

1. Introduction

Care processes are becoming increasingly complex with the growth of technological, biological, and genetic knowledge [1]. This leads naturally to a subdivision of medical specialties, with increasing patient's care costs. Such subdivision, in view of the multiplicity of pathologies of certain patients, complicates diagnosis coding measures, regardless of the coding plan used in clinical and medical-economic settings. It was assumed that incorrect coding of medical information caused, on average, a 14.7% hospital revenue loss per patient [2]. More than three-quarters of these errors are caused by clinicians. These numbers are explained by the intricacy of the classifications and nomenclatures used to code medical acts [3]. In addition, they make it difficult for medical officers to understand the process involved in the coding of this activity [4]. In this context, the establishment of clinical information systems in hospitals can be a key factor in optimizing the coding process of medical information and therefore the expenses of healthcare. The successful establishment of the latter is not done without challenge. In fact, its deployment is based on the data warehouse, which plays an important role in the collection and analysis of large volume of data for decision support. Generally, a data warehouse is often implanted under the relational database management systems (DBMS). The latter obtrudes itself by the richness of their functionality and performance of their request. Nevertheless, they are inadequate to build distributed data warehouses and needful to cope with the scalability of storage space and the increase of hospital stay data [5]. In addition, execution of decision requests demeans the performance of data warehouses in DBMS [6]. In the context of the Georges Pompidou European Hospital, the data warehouse is rapidly growing and contains structured (ICD-10 code, etc.) and unstructured (natural language text, etc.) data of stays from different medical specialties. These data are scattered and do not offer direct access to the medical act coding data based on hierarchies of the 10th revision of International Classification of Disease (ICD-10) for diagnostics as well as the French Common Classification of Medical Act (CCMA) for medical procedures. Moreover, the complexity of the classification in a coding process poses a major problem for sub coding (code forgotten) and over coding (addition of codes not justified) of hospital stays [7]. These challenges can be addressed by providing physicians with a big data storage environment dedicated to coding hospital stays whose particularity is to combine their size (volume), frequency of updates (velocity), or diversity (variety) [8]. Volume, variety, and velocity, often referred to as the three Vs, capture the real meaning of big data [9].

Because big data bring many attractive opportunities to knowledge management [9, 10], the aim of this study is to model the coding data of hospital stays extracted from a data warehouse and implement them in a document-oriented NoSQL data model capable of storing a large distributed big data set. This study sought also to design a big data-coding warehouse efficient for medical coding according to a NoSQL document-oriented data model, which will allow to obtain the optimal combination of codes (diagnoses and acts) for any given reason for care.

2. Methods

This section describes the methodology used to design, implement, and evaluate our data model. Generally, there is a need for a semantic data model to define how data will be structured and related in the database [11], and it is generally acquired that Unified Modeling Language (UML) meets this requirement [12]. Therefore, we first used the formalism of UML [13, 14] to build a conceptual model describing big data of hospital stays. Then, the corresponding rules were used to convert the conceptual model to NoSQL database. In this paper, we choose to focus on document-oriented NoSQL model, namely, MongoDB. This model developed since 2007 by the company of the same name is considered to be the most efficient in terms of performance, for multi-criteria access queries. Finally, the document-oriented model of the big data warehouse was described in JavaScript Object Notation (JSON) format and implemented in the MongoDB database. Subsequently, decision requests were used to evaluate the model.

2.1 Data source

The CIS grouping software for Georges Pompidou European Hospital was used to extract the base of hospital summary report (HSR) from the digestive, oncologic, and orthopedic surgery units. This base of HSR contains a year of hospital stays coded and validated by the department of medical information. Each HSR has medical benefit entities and temporal and administrative patients' data. The entity of medical benefits represented by the medical act and diagnostics appears in three different types of diagnoses: the associated significant diagnosis (ASD), principal diagnosis (PD), and related diagnosis (RD). Moreover, there are various types of acts such as a surgery act and medical technical act.

2.2 Conceptual data model

The goal of a document-oriented database is the representation of more or less complex information that satisfies the needs of flexibility, richness of structure, etc. Modeling of a big data-coding warehouse is a function of the hospital stay's structuring elements. The hospital stay is a document represented by a pair (key, value) and has a tree-shaped structure. The stay entity is the root of the tree. The entities (key) and values for coming up with a conceptual model (**Figure 1**) were designed from the base of HSR. The main entities were defined as an object class that consisted of stay, patient, movement of the patient between the different clinical unit entities, and terminology. The medical benefit entity is a sub-document of stay entities in which the related act and diagnosis are sub-entities.

The entities have a heterogeneous structure and multiple values. The relationship between them is of cardinality "n,m." To ensure that they are unified, it is important to have a flexible open data schema whose structure can be extensible and is able to adapt to more or less important variations. The rank of medical acts, as well as the rank of diagnoses, can easily complete the corresponding type of diagnosis and acts. The rule used to convert the conceptual model to a document-based model is based on the tree model so that the code associates the structure (the tree) and the content (the text in the sheets).

2.3 Correspondence rules with the conceptual/logical level

The coding data are arranged in rows and columns through the big data warehouse model. It is structured into the nested documents in document-oriented NoSQL. The entity stay is a set of facts (patient, movement, medical benefit, etc.) where an instance turns into a nested document. Every sub-entity (movement, medical benefit, etc.) is changed into a nested document. Every sub-sub-entity (Diag, Act, etc.) is changed into a nested document. Every entity also changes to a nested document held in the same document as the fact instance. A stay that has only one main diagnosis is converted into a document that is turned into only one sub-entity Diag. The attributes (key, values) of the other sub-entities are null. There is no preservation of hierarchical organization.

2.4 Document-based model

Under the prism of rules published in Section 2.3, the document-oriented model considers each hospital stay as a key associated with a value. The values can be either

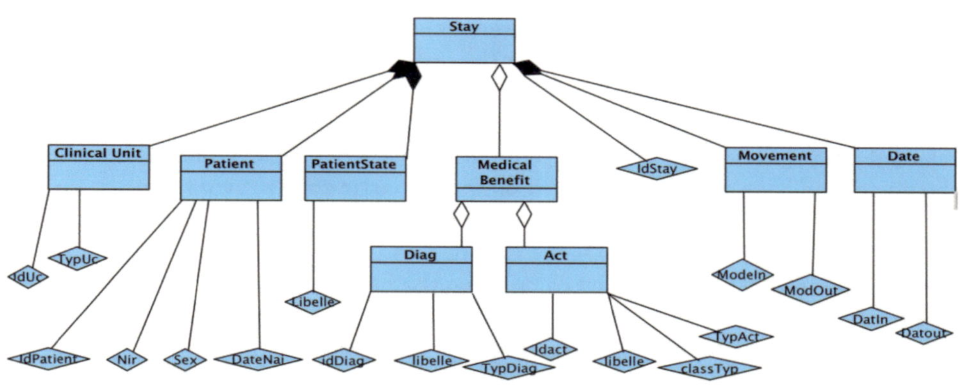

Figure 1.
Hospital stay conceptual data model.

```
{
  "_id": "stay:17",
  "year": "1994",
      "hsr": { "idstay": "4589632" },
      "patient":  { "idpatient": "1236598"},
       "diag": [{ "codediag": "Z092", "typediag":pd"},
                  { "codediag": "N45", "typediag": "rd" },
                  { "codediag": "R589",  "typediag": "asd" },]
        "act": [{"codeact": "ddml556", "typecode": "ATMt1"}
      .... ]
}
{....}
```

Figure 2.
Document-based schema.

atomic value (date of stay) or other documents (patient, medical benefit, etc.). The base of HSRs is a collection of hospital stays, and every stay corresponds to a single entry of this base. The collection includes documents for certain entities, shown through their structure, such as name of the key (medical unit, patients, etc.) and its content (values of the keys (integer (id stay), string (patients, ICD-10), etc.)). The rest of the entities are shown through structural imbrications, such as the medical benefit that is a medical act value aggregate. The entities "medical benefits" refer to an aggregate of a key (diag), which is also an aggregate of (value is ICD-10 code, key is codediag). A document can be defined as a hierarchy of elements that can act as atomic values or nested documents shown by a new set of pairs (value, attribute). There is a simple attribute in the HSR, which makes these values to atomic. The values of compounded attributes are nested documents, as shown in **Figure 2**.

The relationship between different entities is translated in the form of nesting. A document model uses the specific NoSQL request language to query in width and depth all entities present in the collection. A multi- and mono-criteria request can be carried out. An example could be as follows: for a given diagnostic and the type of diagnostic, give all associated diagnostic codes and act codes.

2.5 Evaluation

To evaluate our model, framework MongoDB was deployed in only one data node. The system resources used were (8Go RAM, processor i5–4 heats 2 Terabytes hard disk). MongoDB is a key-value system using document-oriented storage. The volume of data received by one node for the test is 1.6 million documents representing 1 year of the hospital stays. The volume of documents can be worm at 40 times the initial volume. These data are divided into two major groups: encoded and rejected data. The interest of the rejected data is to expand the database, introduce the noise, and have a case of associations of diagnostic code to avoid. Two evaluations were performed. The first one was performed by calculating the model performance (multi-criteria request (Query #2), mono's (Query #1) elapsed time), and the second one was performed by calculating the precision and recall of the model. The initial step was to create two main groups of requests arranged by dimensionality and selectivity validated by the business process, which can be used in a real context. Dimensionality is the value of different keys of the entities ("typediag" and/or "typeact"). Selectivity refers to the degree of data elimination through an aggregate function on the search attribute (code = "CCMA code or ICD-10 code").

Query #1 is expressed as follows: for a given diagnosis or act codes, find all associated code and their corresponding type (typediag, typeact). Three functional use cases were used. The first one concerns the specific case of Z codes as part of the entire ICD-10 code set. Z codes are diagnosis codes used for situations where patients Do not have a known disorder and required a related code to precise the real medical. The second one concerns the code of another chapter of ICD-10, and the last concerns the CCMA act code. Query #2 is expressed as follows: for a given diagnosis and act codes, find all associated codes and their corresponding type (typediag, typeact). Second, through cross-validation, random evaluation is used in measuring the impact of a distributed data storage device on medical procedures' coding optimization. This method provides an opportunity for inserting the process of selection codes of medical acts in a random draw. There are two groups that arise from this draw: an oriented test group with 20% sampling size and 50% of the volume of the data warehouse. The second is a control group with a 50% sampling size and 80% of the data warehouse volume of coding derived by the medical information department. Ten samplings with the same percentage were generated to perform the tests. We used the request previously described to compute the precision and recall of the model. Precision is the ratio between the number of correct associations and the total number of associations, and the ratio is the number of correct associations to the number of all associations to be corrected.

3. Results

The document-oriented model of the big data-coding warehouse was implemented in the MongoDB database. Ten separate single-criteria queries were executed with an elapsed time between 75 and 90 milliseconds (ms), while an elapsed time between 80 and 110 ms was obtained during the execution of 10 separate multi-criteria queries.

Query #1 requests the data warehouse to display all association codes, in which the diagnosis code is equal to "Z092" in the ICD-10 coding system, corresponding to "the pharmacotherapy for other conditions." Associated codes obtained are the associated diagnostic code "E780" used to code "pure hypercholesterolemia" and the act code "EBQM002" used to code "Doppler ultrasonography of extracranial cervicocephalic arteries, with Doppler ultrasound of lower extremity arteries." The elapsed time of this request is 90 ms (**Table 1**).

Table 1 presents results of five sequences of request of Query #1 where requested code represents the code to be queried, associated code represents the obtained associated codes, typology represents different types of diagnostic, and elapsed time represents the execution time of request.

Query #2 requests the data warehouse to display all association codes, in which the type of diagnosis is the main diagnosis and the diagnosis code is equal to "I51.4" in the ICD-10 coding system, corresponding to "cardiomegaly." The response time obtained with no index is approximately 1900 ms. The response time obtained with a diagnostic code indexed is approximately 110 ms. The associated codes are "I080" corresponding to "disorders of mitral and aortic valves" and "D721" corresponding to "eosinophilia," and associated act is "DEQP003" corresponding to "electrocardiography at least 12 leads" (**Table 2**).

Table 2 presents results of five sequences of request of Query #2 where requested code represents the code to be queried and its typologies, associated code represents obtained associated codes (diagnostic and act), typology represents different types of diagnostic, and elapsed time represents the execution time of request.

Requested code	Associated code	Typology	Elapsed time (ms)
I49.9	Not associated code	No typology	75
Z09.8	D35.0	(PD, RD) or (PD, ASD)	85
Z09.8	EBQM002, E78.0	PD, RD, ASD	90
E660.0	I10, N17.9	PD, RD, ASD	87
DEQP003	Z864, I708, E70.8	ACT, PD, RD, ASD	90

Table 1.
Associations of diagnosis codes according to their typology and their elapsed time.

Requested code/typology	Associated code	Typology	Elapsed time (ms)
I49.9/dp	Not associated code	No typology	75
Z09.8/dp	Q21.3	(PD, RD) or (PD, ASD)	85
(Z09.8/dp) and (N185/das)	Z992.1, D638, and JVJB001	PD, RD, and ASD	89
E26.0/dr	Z71.3, D35.0, and DZQM006	PD, RD, ASD, and/or ACT	87
EQQP008	N18.5, I70.2, and Z098	ACT, PD, RD, and ASD	

Table 2.
Associations of diagnosis codes according to their typology and their elapsed time.

Learn/control DB (%)	Precision (%)	Recall (%)
Mono-criteria 50/50	40	25
Mono-criteria 80/20	92	87
Multi-criteria 80/20	80	70

Table 3.
Evaluation results of the big data model.

The list of associated codes present in **Tables 1** and **2** is not exhaustive; it can be extended to more than 100. We make the choice to present a small number.

These results show that the main coding rules have been respected. The associated diagnosis must always be coupled to Z code declared as the main diagnostic and associated acts linked to disease declared as main diagnostic. The presence of related diagnostic demonstrates the quality of associated code containing in the data warehouse.

Query #1 and Query #2 were used to compute the precision and the robustness of the model (**Table 3**).

Based on the observation, the least selective (more lines selected) queries required a long execution time. According to our evaluation, we observed that the system is bijective and corresponds to the reality of the coding of clinical activity of HEGP. This suggests that we can, from the document-oriented model, recover the initial encoding data and vice versa. In this regard, it is apparent that everything that has been set in the big data warehouse corresponds to the reality of the patient. The data warehouse gives the possibility of being more aware of the coding performed in the previous year.

Based on the requests defined above and executed using the learn/control database, **Table 1** shows the results of the evaluation provided by the big data model. The 50/50% precision test was 40 and 25% for recall versus 92/87% for the mono-criteria (Query #1) request. For the multi-criteria (Query #2) request, it was 80/70% for the 80/20% test. Although there are some errors in the test, the sensitivity of conformity computation was 0.8, and its specification was 0.7. Based on this result, the level of accuracy depended on the number of associated diagnostic codes present in the association of codes.

4. Discussion and conclusion

This study investigated the process for implementation of a big data-coding warehouse for coding support in a document-oriented NoSQL system. We observed that flexibility is the particularity of this model as it allows inserting redundancy into the database. A stay with four ASD codes and one PD code is split into four documents. The duplicated line is high when there are more associated diagnoses and medical acts. Therefore, presenting one entity is easier in the entire document. The case of "stay" with only a primary diagnosis, one or more associated diagnosis, and/or without a medical act can be easily inserted in the database without the need to implement a generic code to replace the missing one. In most cases, the addition of a generic code is meant to let the physician understand that there is no need of associating a diagnostic code used with the medical act. This system is advantageous since there is complete information because the issue of missing data is solved. Therefore, the information can be handled without any need to join. Only one reading is needed to get all information. If there is no link between the documents, it is possible to arrange the collection without any challenge. This is an essential part of the construction of a big data-coding warehouse. However, one of the disadvantages associated with this model is that the hierarchization of access does not allow access to ICD-10 code information without going through the type of medical benefit, in addition to the redundancy; there are two pseudorandom choices that provide effective results, while the hazardous choice (50/50%) produces wrong results. To generate huge volumes of data, we used the same "HSR base" and swapped the name ICD-10 by the concept "Obicd10" and CCMA by the concept "Obccam" (Ob as rejected). The rejected data were used to show that, in the optimization process of coding, we learn about as many accepted cases as rejected cases. The major interest in building the coding aid data warehouse is to use the huge volumes of coding information from a large number of hospitals because it is more exhaustive. The model that was implemented allows obtaining an optimal combination of codes (diagnosis, acts) for a given reason for care. Because of the way they are structured, relational databases usually scale vertically—a single server has to host the entire database to ensure reliability and continuous availability of data. This gets expensive quickly, places limits on scale, and creates a relatively small number of failure points for database infrastructure. It's why we propose our model to solve this problem. Indeed, our coding aid data warehouse scales horizontally—several servers host the entire database, allow grouping of all the relevant data for the diagnosis and medical coding in a generic way, to enrich the coding data by crossing the coding information from other hospital sources and to allow for easier exploration of the coding code associations. It's a system that is subject to expertise. This fact Does not remove the richness of Clinical Data Warehouse (CDW). Our contribution consists of building a specific CDW-based document to propose an "in silico" test framework to enhance the efficacy of algorithms used to optimize coding as an example of algorithm based on manual decision-making paper [15] and various natural language processing (NLP) tools associated with the EHR in–/outpatient summary reports [16].

Author details

Joseph Noussa-Yao[1,2]*, Didier Heudes[1,3] and Patrice Degoulet[1,3]

1 INSERM, UMR_S 1138, Paris, France

2 Pierre and Marie Curie University, Paris, France

3 European Hospital Georges Pompidou, France

*Address all correspondence to: jnoussa@gmail.com

References

[1] Ralston JD, Larson EB. Crossing to safety: T ransforming healthcare organizations for patient safety. Journal of Postgraduate Medicine. 2005;**51**(1):61-67

[2] Nouraei SA, O'Hanlon S, Butler CR, Hadovsky A, Donald E, Benjamin E, et al. A multidisciplinary audit of clinical coding accuracy in otolaryngology: Financial, managerial and clinical governance considerations under payment-by-results. Clinical Otolaryngology. 2009;**34**(3):259-260

[3] O'Malley KJ, Cook KF, et al. Measuring diagnoses: ICD code accuracy. Health Services Research. 2005;**40**(5 Part II):1620-1639. DOI: 10.1111/j.1475-6773.2005.00444.x

[4] Puentes J, Montagner J, Lecornu L, Cauvin JM. Information quality measurement of medical encoding support based on usability. Computer Methods and Programs in Biomedicine. 2013;**112**:329-342

[5] Leavitt N. Will nosql database live up to their promise? Computer. 2010;**43**(2):12-14

[6] Golfarelli M, Maio D, Rizzi S. The dimensional fact model: A conceptual model for data warehouses. International Journal of Cooperative Information Systems. 1998;**7**:215-247

[7] Chaudhuri S, Dayal U. An overview of data warehousing and OLAP technology. ACM Sigmod Record. 1997;**26**:65-74

[8] Hay SI, George DB, Moyes CL, Brownstein JS. Big Data opportunities for global infectious disease surveillance. PLoS Medicine. 2013;**10**(4):e1001413. DOI: 10.1371/journal.pmed.1001413

[9] Chen CP, Zhang CY. Data-intensive applications, challenges, techniques and technologies: A survey on Big Data. Information Sciences. 2014;**275**:314-347. DOI:10.1016/j.ins.2014.01.015

[10] Fredriksson C. Knowledge management with big-data creating new possibilities for organizations. In: The XXIVth Nordic Local Government Research Conference (NORKOM); Gothenburg: Nordiska kommunforskarkonferensen; 2015

[11] Daniel G, Sunyé G, Cabot J. UML to graph DB: Mapping conceptual schemas to graph databases. In: Comyn-Wattiau I, Tanaka K, Song IY, Yamamoto S, Saeki M. editors. Conceptual Modeling. Vol. 9974. Springer, Cham.: Lecture Notes in Computer Science; 2016. https://doi.org/10.1007/978-3-319-46397-1_33

[12] Abadi D, Boncz P, Harizopoulos S, Idreos S, Madden S. The design and implementation of modern column-oriented database systems. Foundations and Trends in Databases. 2013;**5**(3):197-280. DOI: 10.1561/1900000024

[13] Object Management Group, Inc. 2005. UML 2.0 Superstructure. Available from: http://www.omg.org/cgi-bin/apps/doc?formal/05-07-04.pdf

[14] Luj'an-Mora S, Trujillo J, Song IY. A UML profile for multidimensional modeling in data warehouses. Data and Knowledge Engineering. 2006;**59**(3):725-769

[15] Lecomu L, Thillay G, Le Guillou C, Garreau PJ, Saliou P, Puentes J, et al. REFEROCOD: A probabilistic method to medical coding support. In: Conference Proceedings: Annual International Conference of the IEEE Engineering in Medicine and Biology Society 2009; 2009. pp. 3421-3424

[16] Mitchell JB, Bubolz T, Paul JE, Pashos CL, Escarce JJ, Muhlbaier LH, et al. Using medicare claims for outcomes research. Medical Care. 1994;**32**(7 Suppl):JS38-JS51